Doreen 90

Self-Massage

Touch Techniques to Relax, Soothe and Stimulate Your Body

by Monika Struna
with Connie Church

Photographs by Trudy Schlachter
Drawings by Sandra Garelick

A Fireside Book
Published by Simon and Schuster
New York

Copyright © 1983 by Monika Struna and Connie Church
All rights reserved
including the right of reproduction
in whole or in part in any form
A Fireside Book
Published by Simon and Schuster
A Division of Gulf & Western Corporation
Simon & Schuster Building
Rockefeller Center
1230 Avenue of the Americas
New York, New York 10020
FIRESIDE and colophon are registered trademarks of Simon & Schuster
Designed by Irving Perkins Associates
Manufactured in the United States of America
Printed and bound by Halliday Lithograph
10 9 8 7 6 5 4 3 2
Library of Congress Cataloging in Publication Data
Struna, Monika.
    Self-massage.

    "A Fireside book."
    1. Massage.   2. Self-care, Health.   I. Church, Connie,
1955–   .   II. Title.
RA780.5.S68   1983   646.7′5   82-19557
ISBN: 0-671-45694-6

Acknowledgments

Special thanks to our agent Susan Zeckendorf for believing in *Self-Massage*. It was her nurturing, patience, and guidance that made this book possible.

Also thanks to Joan Katz and Curt Struna for helping me get started; and to Kathleen Brimlow, Roberta Wein, physical therapist, David Goldman, D.C., Debbie Sherman, M.D., Lindy Ferigno, and Annie Roget for their helpful suggestions; and to Paul Diner, photographer, for taking a chance. Special last-minute thanks to Dr. Ernest April and Maureen Heffernan and Charles Rue Woods, our editors.

Thanks to Allen and to our families, who gave us emotional and financial support when it was needed.

Finally, thanks to our numerous friends whose confidence and sharing of experience played so large a part.

*I wish to thank all the people I've worked
with over the years who came to me for guidance
in self-help. Their requests for this information
inspired me to do this book and sustained me
throughout its development.*

Monika Struna

Contents

Contents

Introduction

HOW MANY times during the day do you endure tension and stress? The kids are screaming, the dinner is burning, the television is blaring, the phone and doorbell ring at the same time, and you have a pounding headache with hours to go before you can sit down and relax. Or, you're at the office and you realize it's three o'clock and you haven't had lunch, the phone has been ringing all day, you've pushed papers in every direction, and you have an important presentation to make to the head of the firm in ten minutes. The pressure is mounting, your neck and shoulders are tense, your stomach is burning from too much coffee, and your expression is anything but relaxed and smiling.

We all experience situations of stress and the pain it causes (and probably in more interesting and original ways than the above). How do we handle it? Run out the door? Jump out a window? Go to Tahiti? Hit the bottle? Probably not. The health boom is on and a great majority of us have made organic foods, an abundance of vitamins, and jogging and exercise a regular part of our lives. Whether we are six or sixty, looking good and feeling good has become a way of life—and a necessary one if we are to function effectively and happily in our frantic, fast-paced society.

But there are some days when we are just too exhausted mentally and physically to go out and run that mile, do those sit-ups and leg lifts, or change our clothes and go to the gym. Or perhaps we are housebound with a sick child, have sprained an ankle, or have some other condition that makes physical exercise impossible. However, we still need a healthy way to unwind, let our hair down, and just plain relax. For this there is self-massage.

And what about those little aches and pains that make us reach for the aspirin bottle or send us running to the doctor? We are usually told that they are stress-induced and that we should learn to relax. And besides leaving us stiff and aching, this excessive tension and stress

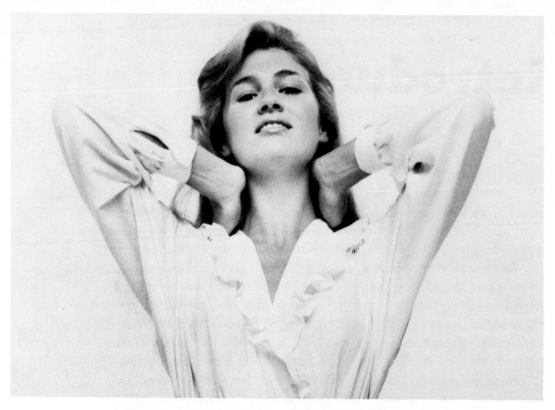

can cause general ill-health within our bodies. Not only do abnormally tight, tense muscles operate ineffectively, but they impede proper circulation as well. When the circulation is impaired, fresh blood is unable to reach and nourish the tissues, and waste products collect. This causes a decreased exchange of fluids within the tissues, leading to fatigue and a general imbalance within our body systems.

The function of the blood capillary systems and the lymphatic system is to maintain and regulate our body's fluid balance. When we are active, fluids are pumped into the muscles (fluids such as blood proteins, water, leukocytes, and fats). Whatever excesses the blood capillary system can't handle, the lymphatic system takes care of. Excessive and chronic tension impedes this fluid exchange and lessens the muscle's ability to contract.

Massage acts as a mechanical cleanser as it increases the interchange of tissue fluids emptied into the blood capillary and lymphatic network, removing the products of fatigue and inflammation. By doing this, massage indirectly increases the tone (the muscle's *normal* state of tension) of the muscles being treated by passively increasing the contracting power of the muscles. While bringing about a deep sense of relaxation, massage also improves circulation, helps maintain fluid balance, and relieves excess tension. Self-massage is a personal way to help maintain your own well-being.

Self-massage is immediately available to everybody—you probably use some form of it already. There is a natural reflex response in us to soothe and alleviate discomfort by touching ourselves. At times of injury a hand automatically goes to the pain. When your head hurts you rub it. When you get a stiff neck you try to massage the stiffness out. You are actually practicing self-massage at home, in your car, at the office, anytime and anywhere. *Self-Massage* shows you how to properly guide and manipulate your instinctively healing hands and fingers. No one knows *you* as well as *you*—where it hurts and what feels good.

Massage is not a new concept. It is the earliest known form of healing —touch—developed over thousands of years and surviving into modern technological society. Almost every culture has employed it, including the Celts, Goths, Egyptians, Greeks, and Romans. It is evident that massage has been with man from the beginning.

The two major and most widely used methods of massage are the Eastern meridian System and the Western Swedish muscular manipulation. It is not important if one is better or more effective, but rather how to use what is available from both.

The Eastern systems derive from Do-In, the oldest known approach to holistic life. Picture Do-In as a huge tree with many branches. Shiatsu (we will refer to it as pressure point therapy), the most recent name given to manually manipulating the points that make up the meridian system, is one branch.

The meridian system is best described as a series of points bilaterally located within the body that may be reached by applying pressure to the skin's surface. When these points are connected they form an invisible channel, also called a line or a pathway. There are fourteen major channels. Some are named after the vital organs whose functions they facilitate—lung, kidney, spleen, small intestines, and so forth— and some are named after the function they regulate—governing vessel (brain), conception vessel (sex), triple heater (circulation, metabolism), and heart constrictor (vascular, protector of the heart). The points are conductors of energy and are in constant flux as they conduct positive and negative charges throughout our bodies and bring about a state of balance in our internal environment. The points themselves may also be called resistors because that is where the energy exchange is most likely to become stagnated and create imbalance. It is this stagnation and eventual imbalance that is believed to be the cause of illness. Pressure therapy is applied as a preventive discipline intended to alleviate energy blocks, thereby stimulating the body's own curative powers.

Swedish massage is a uniquely Western interpretation of massage, but with roots in ancient Eastern cultures. It is the most popular and widely used system in this country, first introduced by Pehr Henrik Ling in 1812. He based his system on the techniques of a Taoist priest, Tao-of-Shinsen, who actively adapted exercises from Do-In. The connection of East and West is obvious, making Swedish massage another branch of the ancient art of manipulation.

Swedish massage stimulates circulation and the nervous system's response. It also helps strengthen muscle and skin tissue while relaxing stressed areas of the body. Although many claim that massage aids in breaking down adipose (fatty) tissue, this has not been clinically proven. But there *are* beautifying effects of massage. Massage indirectly improves muscle tone and stimulates the circulatory system, leaving you with glowing, healthy skin. Massage combined with proper diet and active exercise can only further enhance your total well-being.

Self-Massage combines the systems of East and West for simplified everyday use: it expands on the natural reflex response and helps you find a quick and easy direction for it. There are no special tools to purchase, diets to follow, or clothing to buy, because self-massage is applied mainly through the use of hands and fingers. Self-massage can be used to stimulate all body systems and has been helpful in treating some forms of arthritis. By performing self-massage a relationship of active and passive experience is created. Receiving the massage is passive exercise while administering the massage is active exercise. Therefore, not only the manipulated area is getting treatment, but also the hand (or whichever part of the body is used) performing the massage or manipulation is actively exercising. This is especially beneficial to arthritics and bedridden patients who have little or no exercise in their lives.

Self-Massage offers a systematic approach to self-healing as well as a chance to create your own beautiful well-being. It is for everyone who has ever felt the need to work with his or her own body: the business executive, the mother on her infant's schedule, the athlete, the elderly, the bedridden. Learning to deal with the physical tension in your body and getting in touch with your body, for yourself by yourself, can only create a better self-image. How often have we all wondered, "What can I do to help myself?" *Self-Massage* offers a therapeutic alternative for dealing with stress, physical tension, and anxiety. With *Self-Massage* you can learn how to unlock untapped energy.

Many people deprive themselves of any massage experience because it is either not accessible, or too expensive. Some stay away from massage out of simple inhibition. I want to touch as many lives as possible by showing you the benefits of touching yourself.

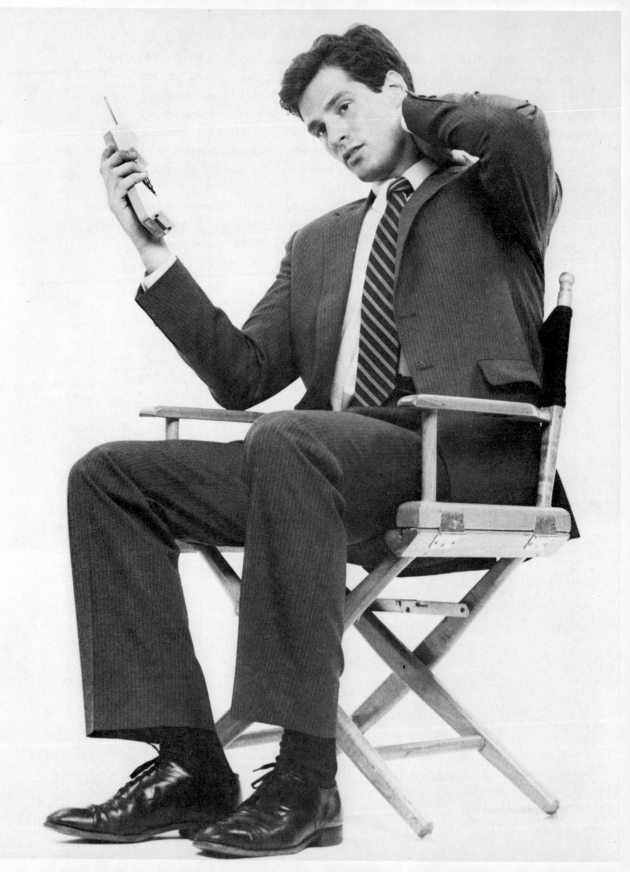

Self-Massage Technique

BEFORE YOU begin working on specific stress sites, read this section carefully. Avoid rushing and doing too much at once. I recommend that you limit working on any one part of the body to ten minutes —especially when localizing treatment and executing the deeper moves. You can always return to the area after a period of rest. Practice each movement until you feel confident with it. The time you spend now will be well worth it. Eventually you will become proficient enough so that the movements will come easily, so when you reach for that aching neck or shoulder your hands will naturally massage it most effectively. When you feel comfortable with the movements, you can create your own personalized full-body massage by choosing one movement for each part of the body from the movements recommended in the following chapters.

As you work out localized areas of tension, listen to your body: be aware of your breath, fingers, thumbs, palms, elbows and recognize their healing potential. Always remember to relax and not to strain. Go with the movement in an unhurried manner, keeping shoulders, neck, and wrists loose. This will help to lessen fatigue. Shake fingers and hands out from time to time to expel any tension which collects. The more relaxed you remain, the greater the effects of your self-massage.

The magic and skill is innate in your hands and comes from a natural integration of breath, mind, and body. The ability to feel better is within you. Go slowly and listen to your body. (A little lower to the right, please!) And enjoy!

Breathing and Relaxing

Not only does breathing keep us alive, it also activates all body mechanics and aids in all of our body functions. The major function of the heart and lungs is to produce and bring oxygen-rich blood to all body tissues. As the tissues are nourished, the mechanics of breathing act as an internal organ massage as well. When you inhale, air is brought into the lungs, the diaphragm descends, the thoracic cavity expands, and the pressure in the abdomen is increased. Exhaling causes the diaphragm to contract into a dome shape and increases the pressure within the thoracic cavity. Exhaling also puts pressure on the blood vessels and lymph tubes so that the fluids move up toward the heart, aiding circulation as it hastens the elimination of waste. As deep breathing helps our heart and lungs to work more effectively it also brings about a deep sense of relaxation, focus, harmony, and center.

When doing self-massage, deep breathing will keep you relaxed and help synchronize the massage movements with your body's natural functioning. And as the pressure and manipulation of your self-massage opens up the circulation, deep breathing will bring nourishing oxygen-rich blood to all body parts.

A Breathing Exercise. This can be done in any position. Begin with a slow deep inhalation through your *nose* to the count of 1-2-3-4-5. The focus is on centering yourself as you bring your breath from the chest to the stomach and then to the abdomen. Place your hands on your navel and feel it distend. Then slowly exhale through the *nose or mouth* to the count of 1-2-3-4-5, feeling the abdomen contract. Visualize your breath with your eyes, hear it with your ears, and feel it throughout your body. Become the breath—nothing more.

Ideally, in doing any self-massage you should be aware of your breathing and try to develop normal deep-breathing patterns. Your body will be more relaxed and receptive to self-massage as you focus on the movements being in harmony with your breathing.

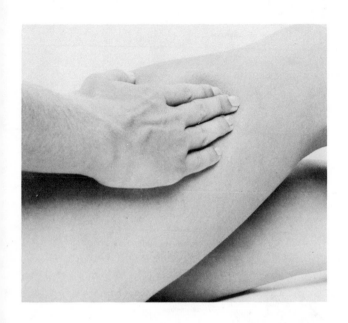
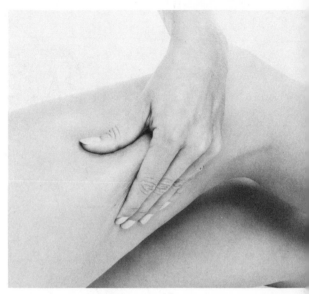

Use the basic techniques given in the following chapter as guidelines to explore the sensitivity of your own body in relation to touch and movement. Once you have discovered the freedom within the movements, you can expand upon them and use them according to your individual needs.

Stroking is used mainly to warm up, soothe, and prepare the body for deeper movements. Traditionally, *stroking* is used before and after other movements to explore and prepare the area for deeper movements. It can be done with the fingers, whole hand, and forearm. The heels of the feet are also good to use when stroking inner and outer legs. Follow the direction of the muscle fibers with long consistent strokes on the skin's surface. *Stroking* can be done with varying degrees of pressure and in a circular motion. Experiment with different amounts of pressure and find what feels good to you. Strokes are to be directed toward the heart, aiding blood flow and the lymphatic system. (*Stroking* is how most of us respond and touch ourselves when we have pain.)

Pinching is just what it sounds like. But it should always be done gently to avoid bruising. For harder *pinching* squeeze tissue between

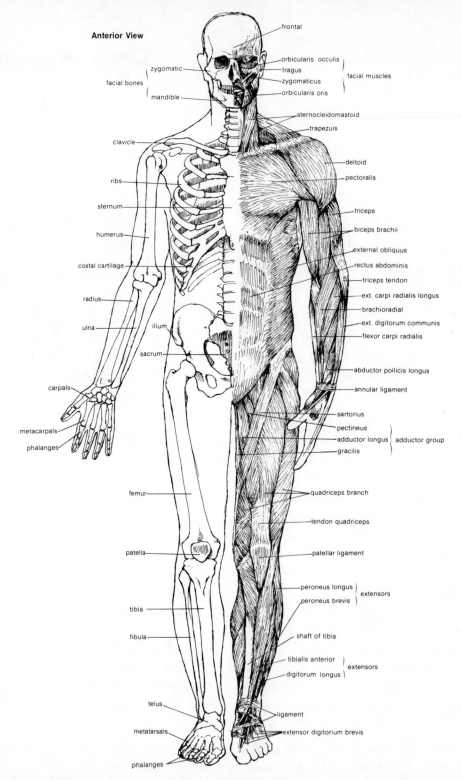

Anterior View

frontal

facial bones
- zygomatic
- mandible

orbicularis occulis
tragus
zygomaticus
orbicularis oris

facial muscles

sternocleidomastoid
trapezuis

clavicle

ribs

sternum

humerus

costal cartilage

radius

ulna

ilium

sacrum

carpals

metacarpals

phalanges

deltoid
pectoralis
triceps
biceps brachii
external obliquus
rectus abdominis
triceps tendon
ext. carpi radialis longus
brachioradial
ext. digitorum communis
flexor carpi radialis

abductor pollicis longus
annular ligament

sartorius
pectineus
adductor longus
gracilis

adductor group

femur

patella

tibia

fibula

quadriceps branch
tendon quadriceps
patellar ligament

peroneus longus
peroneus brevis

extensors

shaft of tibia

tibialis anterior
digitorum longus

extensors

telus

metatarsals

phalanges

ligament
extensor digitorium brevis

This illustration shows the direction of the superior muscle fibers located within
the individual muscle groups and their underlying bony structure. When you mas-

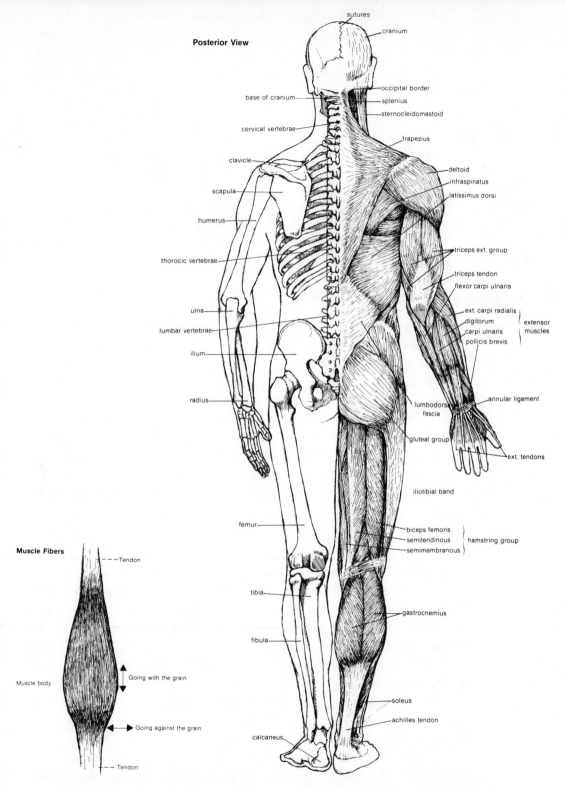

Posterior View

sutures

cranium

base of cranium

occipital border

splenius

sternocleidomastoid

cervical vertebrae

trapezius

clavicle

deltoid

infraspinatus

latissimus dorsi

scapula

humerus

triceps ext. group

triceps tendon

flexor carpi ulnaris

thorocic vertebrae

ext. carpi radialis

digitorum

ulna

carpi ulnaris

extensor
muscles

lumbar vertebrae

pollicis brevis

ilium

radius

annular ligament

lumbodorsi
fascia

gluteal group

ext. tendons

iliotibial band

femur

biceps femoris

semitendinous

semimembranous

hamstring group

tibia

gastrocnemius

fibula

Muscle Fibers

Tendon

Muscle body

Going with the grain

Going against the grain

Tendon

soleus

achilles tendon

calcaneus

sage, you will either be working along or against the grain of the muscle fiber.

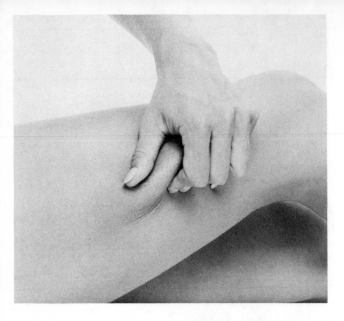
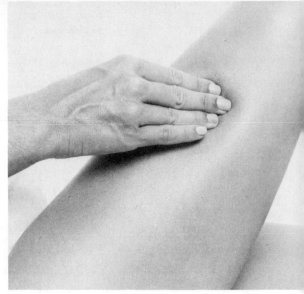

the fingers. For lighter *pinching* squeeze the tissue between palm and fingers, pulling muscle tissue slightly away from the bone. *Pinching* is effective in improving circulation and stimulating sluggish muscles.

Rolling is best described as a light pinch gliding along the skin's surface without breaking contact. It is done with or against the grain of muscle fibers. Lift up, pulling away from the bone, and slightly pinch the tissue. Let the thumb give support and drag while the fingers walk and roll the muscle. It can be done with one hand or with two hands side by side, and is good to use when working with smaller muscle groups. Rolling stimulates circulation and passively strengthens weak muscles.

Friction movements are best done with four fingers, but can be done with just the thumb or the palm of the hand. They are circular movements that go deep into the muscle—not just surface rubbing. Apply fingers with moderate to deep pressure and actively separate muscle fibers as you make circles with a relaxed, rhythmic motion. Use your fingers for making small circles and your whole hand for larger ones. Elbows and forearms are also good to use when making larger circles (especially on legs and thighs). *Friction* is especially good to use around joints, shoulder blades, and the soles of the feet because it stretches tendons and ligaments. It is also effective in breaking down scar tissue and waste deposits. Friction movements stimulate circulation and metabolic interchange.

Percussion movements are striking, slicing, hacking, chopping movements done in a rapid rhythmic motion. They are used mostly on the

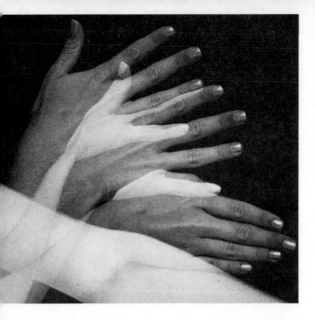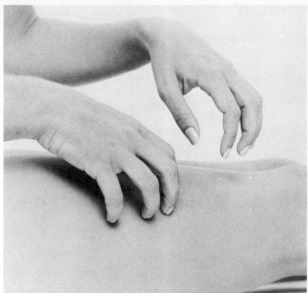

fleshier parts of the body and serve to stimulate nerve endings and the circulatory system, dispersing metabolic waste products. You can use one hand or alternate both hands. Remember always to keep your wrists loose. The *percussion* movements are broken down into the following categories:

Slapping is done with an open hand and the flat surface of the fingers. It can be used on all body parts. Start with the head and work downward, alternating your hands in a rhythmic motion.

Hacking is the massage movement seen on television and in the movies. It is done with the pinkie side of the hand (or outer edge of the palm of the hand) and can be done hard or soft:

Hard Hacking: Fingers should be held *together* and kept relaxed as body contact is made with the outer edge of the palm. Alternate hands with a slicing rhythmic motion.

Soft Hacking: Keep fingers slightly *separated* and relaxed. As the pinkie finger strikes, the other fingers will follow naturally.

Tapping can be done with the tips of the fingers if nail length permits. Separating the fingers slightly, apply alternating strokes to the fleshier parts of the body.

Cupping is done with fingers held together in a half fist. (The hand should look like a cup.) A suction noise will be created on con-

Self-Massage Technique

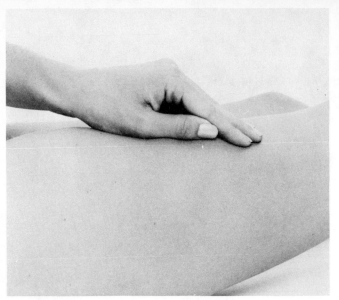
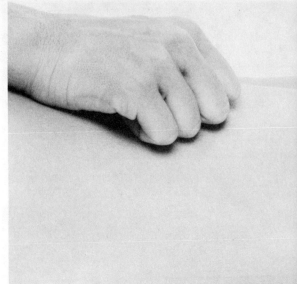

tact. When applied to the chest and rib cage, cupping can be effective in loosening mucous membranes and relieving bronchial congestion.

All of the *percussion* movements should be executed firmly and strongly, but should never be painful. Be careful not to bruise or rupture the capillary network beneath the surface of the skin. Avoid performing any of these movements on bone protuberances, glands, or on the abdominal region.

Knuckles can be applied to the body by stroking or in light striking motions. With a relaxed fist and wrist, body contact is made with the second phalange (joint space) of fingers.

Vibration is just what it sounds like and may seem a little difficult to perform at first—but it is well worth learning. It is important that you remember to keep the shoulders and neck relaxed at all times. Executed with the fingers or the palm of the hand, *vibration* is best described as a rapid shaking or trembling movement on the skin's surface without breaking contact. There are a few variations of this movement:

> *Vertical vibration* is stationary *vibration* moving up and down on the skin's surface without breaking contact.
> *Horizontal vibration* is stationary *vibration* moving sideways on

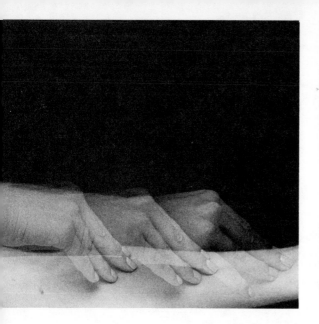
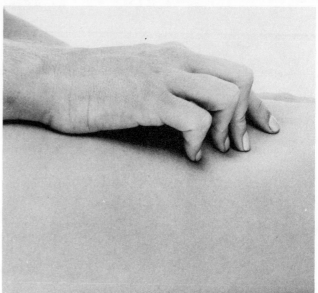

the skin's surface without breaking contact.

Running vibration is any of the *vibration* movements used while gliding along the skin's surface. The pressure should be deep while the moving hand continuously vibrates.

While using any *vibration* it is suggested that you vibrate 3 seconds and rest 2 seconds. As you practice, the rhythm will become natural. If the hands are weak, one hand can be placed over the other for support. *Vibration* is effective in stimulating local nerve response, loosening stiff joints and stretching scar tissue. When applied to abdominal regions it stimulates peristalsis. *Vibration* is also very soothing and relaxing.

Raking is one of the easier movements that can be done on almost any part of the body. It is especially good on the neck and the larger muscle groups. Raking is best applied by going against the grain of muscle fibers. Deep contact is made by hooking the finger tips into the soft tissue while pulling and gliding along the skin's surface. A variation of this movement is done by alternating your fingers in any order while pulling them toward the palm of the hand. The palm should be anchored in a stationary position for leverage and support. This movement works best when the muscle is not contracted, so relax and enjoy its warming effects.

Self-Massage Technique

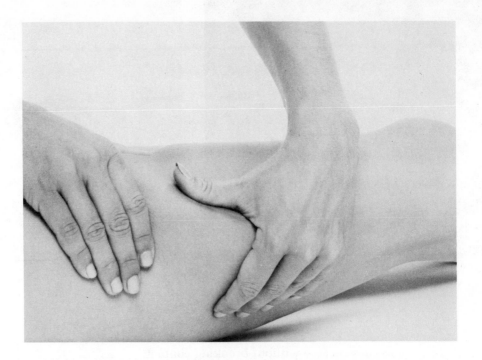

Petrissage is the classic word for the rhythmic kneading of a muscle. It is a progressive picking up and rolling pressing movement as you push with one hand and pull with the other in an alternating pattern. The hands should glide vertically along the muscle body without breaking contact. *Petrissage* is especially good for the bedridden, as it helps prevent atrophy by stretching and strengthening the muscle. It helps to remove waste products as it increases the circulation and indirectly tones the muscles.

Centering is establishing a point of focus, allowing the movements to come naturally and without effort. It is an integral part of massage that underlies every technique. Centering is accomplished through concentration and breath: be still, relax, focus your attention on your breath, and wait as you feel yourself calming. Having this centered feeling allows you to move with purpose and without strain.

Holding is the most natural response to pain. It is a calming technique that soothes the nerve response of an injured area. *Hold* the pain by supporting the area with the palm and fingers of one or two hands or just use one or two fingers. Center your breath as you *hold*. Listen and wait for the *pulse*. Throughout our bodies there are electromagnetic fields which conduct positive and negative energy. *Holding* until

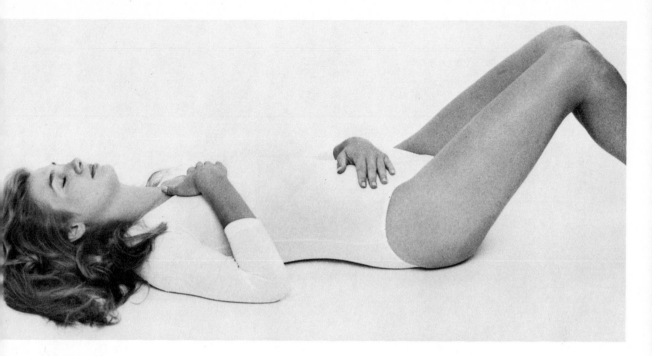

you feel a pulse frees the injured area of any energy blocks that may have occurred. *Holding* is the best way to release the body's own wonderful healing mechanisms. As you *hold,* jiggling a bit will help the pulse pop in. You can hold a point for as long as 20 minutes. Just touch, listen, and feel.

Pressure Therapy. When you perform Pressure Therapy, you are stimulating the points which make up the meridian channels. The general location of all points is illustrated in the chart on pp. 30–31. However, the location of the points may vary slightly in each person. Feel for individual points as they are more sensitive to the touch. Pressure is applied in order to release energy blocks within these channels. By stimulating the points the circulation is improved throughout all body systems, helping to maintain energy balance and general good health. The traditional numbering corresponds to the direction of energy flow within each meridian channel. Directions on how to use this system are to be given in the following chapters.

Stationary vertical pressure means applying pressure without movement at a 90° angle to the contour of the body's surface. It is best applied with the thumbs. You can also experiment with the palms, elbows, and heels of the feet for more general treatment. When using the thumb (no fingernails, please!), light pressure is applied with the

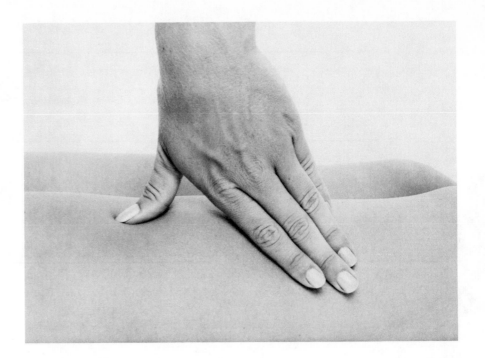

ball of the thumb and hard pressure is applied with the tip. By using your four fingers for support and leverage and moving your wrist or elbow, you can regulate the degree of intensity. Elbows are good for applying pressure therapy because you can use your weight and lean into your body to achieve different amounts of pressure. Deeper penetration will come naturally as you hold the point longer. Pressure is applied gradually, and the point should be held until stimulation is felt. If nothing is felt, try changing the degree of the angle. When you feel the change, hold briefly and then move on to the next point. (Meridien charts illustrate specific points.)

Pressure therapy. Some basics first. When applying pressure therapy remember that the center of gravity is below your navel and your breath is the energy. Pressure therapy should be effortless. Use your body weight whenever possible, rather than muscle; *lean* into the points being affected instead of pushing. Follow the meridian lines, as illustrated in the chart, affecting the beginning and the end of the channel on both sides of the body. Bring your breath into motion by synchronizing the movements with your breathing. Exhale as you lean into points applying pressure, inhale as you release.

SELF-MASSAGE

STATIONARY VERTICAL PRESSURE

Elbows

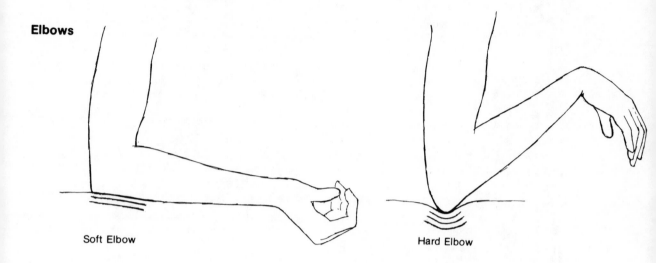

Soft Elbow

Hard Elbow

Thumbs

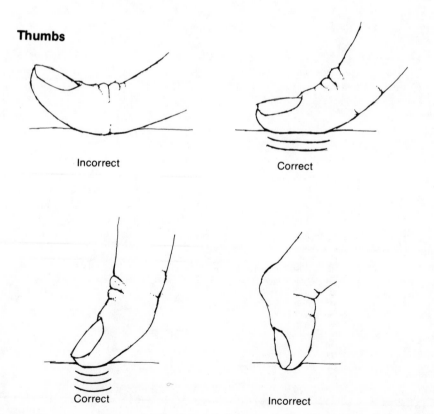

Incorrect

Correct

Correct

Incorrect

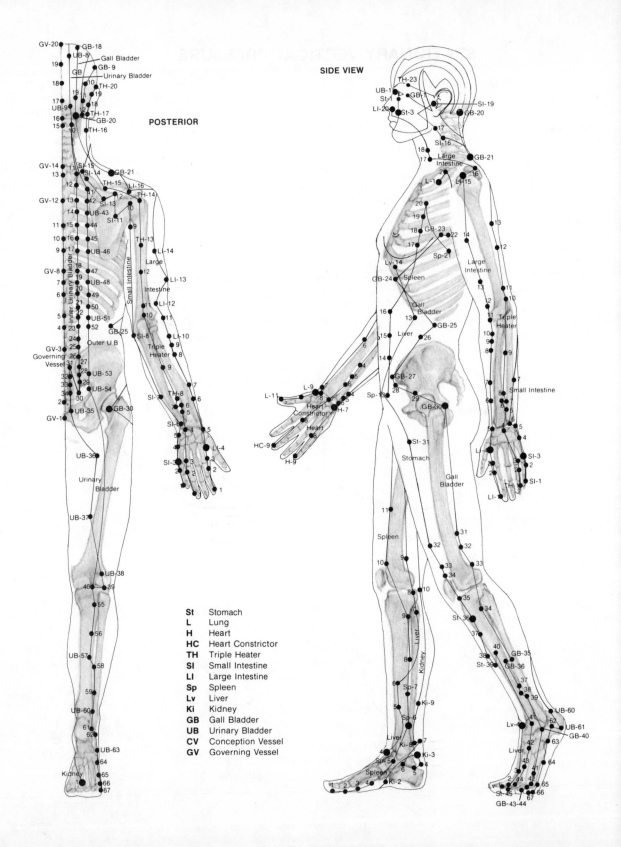

POSTERIOR

SIDE VIEW

St Stomach
L Lung
H Heart
HC Heart Constrictor
TH Triple Heater
SI Small Intestine
LI Large Intestine
Sp Spleen
Lv Liver
Ki Kidney
GB Gall Bladder
UB Urinary Bladder
CV Conception Vessel
GV Governing Vessel

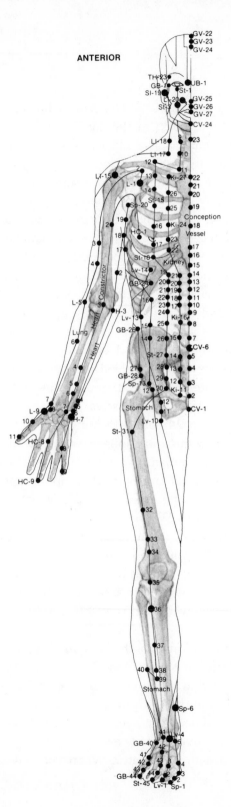

Meridian Chart

The illustrations show the traditional numbering and location of the points on the meridian channels. Points are numbered to indicate the direction of the flow of energy within each channel. Directions on how to perform pressure therapy on specific areas of the body are given in the following chapters.

Follow the meridian lines as they are illustrated here. Remember to synchronize your movements with your breath.

Household
Helpers

You need nothing for self-massage but yourself. This means that you can treat those tense trouble spots at work, in the car—anywhere! However, in your home there are many household helpers. As you explore and become adept with the basic self-massage techniques you may wish to expand with accessories. The following are some of the household helpers with which you may wish to experiment.

Towels. A simple bath towel when folded correctly can be used to apply pressure to those hard-to-reach spots. It can also be used to make hot and cold packs which can be applied to stiff or spasmodic muscles.

Hot packs. There are many ways to apply hot packs, from soaking a towel to using hot water bags. Hot packs are not to be applied for at least 24 hours after acute injury, and when used are only applied at 20-minute intervals. Dry heat is not as effective as moist heat on muscles and is often overused. Moist heat goes deep into muscles, dilating blood vessels, allowing for oxygen-rich blood to nourish the tissues. This provides for metabolic interchange and promotes healing. Moist heat is recommended for tense, tight, stiff muscles.

Cold packs. Ice is applied for the first 24 hours after an acute muscular injury at 20-minute intervals to minimize inflammation by increasing the absorption of excess inflammatory exudates. It is also effective in relieving muscular tension and stiffness when applied at 10-minute intervals. By applying cold to the stress site you slow activity, allowing muscles and nerves to rest. When the cold pack is removed the blood vessels dilate rapidly, warming up the area and bringing in fresh oxygenated blood. This increases the interchange of tissue fluids and promotes healing. Try putting a wet towel in the freezer until it is iced. You may want to wrap it in saran wrap to keep it from sticking to the freezer. A frozen wet towel is effective on those tense shoulders and stiff necks.

Bathing. Water has the power to heal and soothe tension. A therapeutic bath cutting off all external stimuli is pure bliss. There are many ways to bathe, but one bath that I find to be especially helpful for stress and tension is the *pack bath*. Fill the tub with the hottest water you can tolerate. Submerge your total body but keep your head above the water. Before you begin to feel overheated, allow the water to drain as you gradually fill the tub with cold water. When you have cooled down, begin again by draining the cold water as you fill the tub with hot water. Repeat the process. When you remove yourself from the tub you will be relaxed as well as invigorated. The cleansing and relaxing *pack bath* works the circulatory system as it contracts and dilates the blood vessels. The tub is a good place to practice self-massage when taking a regular warm bath. Adding salts, oils, and scents will also enhance your bathing experience.

Contraindications

As with any other self-help therapy, there are times when self-massage should not be done. If you are suffering from any severe medical conditions, taking any prescriptions, or have any doubts about using any of the techniques, consult your physician first. These applications are not for treatment of any pathological disorders.

Do not massage when there is an indication of:

1. Disease of bones, muscles, skin (example: dermatomyositis)
2. Virus
3. Unhealed fractures. After the bone has healed you may massage the fracture site.
4. Unhealed acutely ruptured muscles
5. Bacterial, acutely inflammatory, or severe localized arthritis
6. Phlebitis or varicose veins
7. Pain due to infection
8. Undiagnosed masses
9. Hemorrhage
10. Vomiting
11. Acute pain in the abdomen. Also, do not massage the abdomen immediately after meals.
12. Unstable cardiac conditions

The Face
and Head

PATTING

Position: Standing with your feet approximately 12 inches apart, using both of your hands.

Application: 1. Lean forward slightly as if you are going to touch your toes, allowing for comfort and balance.
2. With both hands use the flat portion of your fingers to vigorously pat the entire face. Pat for 15 to 20 seconds.

Beneficial Effects: Feel the warm glow spread across your face as you bring circulation to the area, stimulating and nourishing the delicate facial skin.

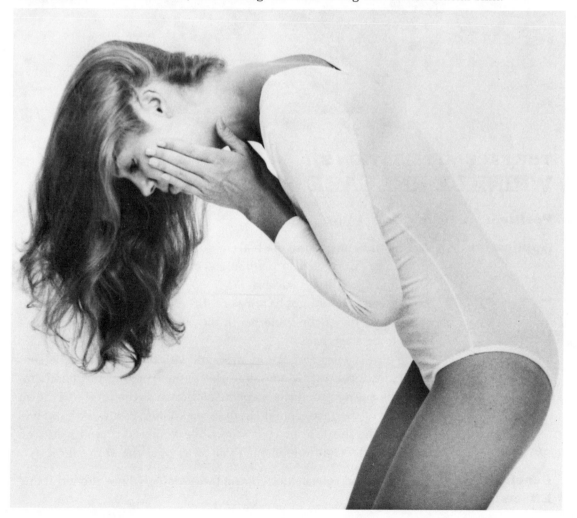

The Face and Head

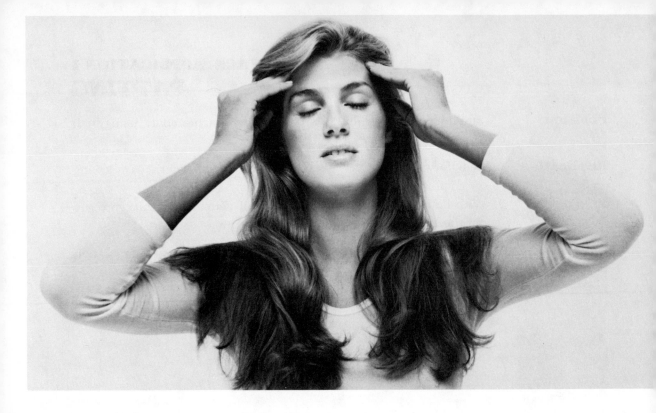

THE FACE: APPLICATION 2
WRINKLE RELEASE

Position: Any, using both of your hands.

Application: 1. With both hands, using the balls of your fingertips, apply moderate to deep pressure as you manipulate back and forth the tissue beneath the facial skin's surface.

2. Your fingers should apply pressure directly into your face. As you manipulate the tissue underneath the skin's surface, the skin itself is not to be stretched.

3. Begin on the forehead. Apply pressure with both hands at the center of the forehead. Manipulate the tissue, moving the hands toward the sides of the face. Repeat. Work across the forehead, down the sides of the face, and along the cheekbones. Your left hand will work on the left side of your face while your right hand works on the right side. Continue inching your way over the entire face.

Beneficial Effects: Nourishes and relaxes underlying facial tissue where the wrinkling process begins.

STROKING THE EARS

Position: Any, using both of your hands.

Application: 1. Using one hand on each side, straddle the base of your ears with your index and middle fingers.
2. With your ears in between your index and middle fingers, stroke your ears by moving your fingers up and down.
3. Stroke 10 to 15 times. This can be repeated as often as you like.

Variation: Try flaring your ears out from your head, using the fingers from each hand. The movement of your hands is from the back to the front as your fingers flip your ears out from your head. Flare 3 to 5 times.

Beneficial Effects: Soothes and warms the ears.
Relaxes the jaw muscles.
Stimulates ear reflexes.

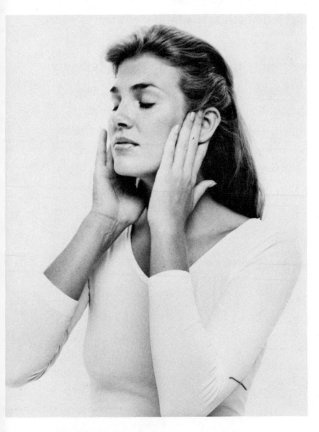
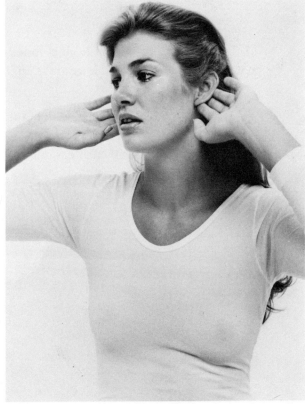

THE FACE: APPLICATION 4
STIMULATING THE EARS

Position: Any, using both of your hands.

Application: *Stretching*

1. Using one hand on each ear, hold the earlobes with your thumb and index finger. Pinch and then slowly pull, *stretching* the ear outward without twisting. Work your way from the lobe up and around the entire edge of the ear. You can do both ears simultaneously.

Pressure

2. Now, with your index finger apply moderate amounts of pressure along the inside border of the ears.

Uncurling

3. Gently *uncurl* the outer folds of the ears. This is the area at the top of the ears.
4. Work each ear once by *stretching*, *pressing*, and *uncurling*.

Beneficial Effects: Stimulates the points and reflexes located on the ear.

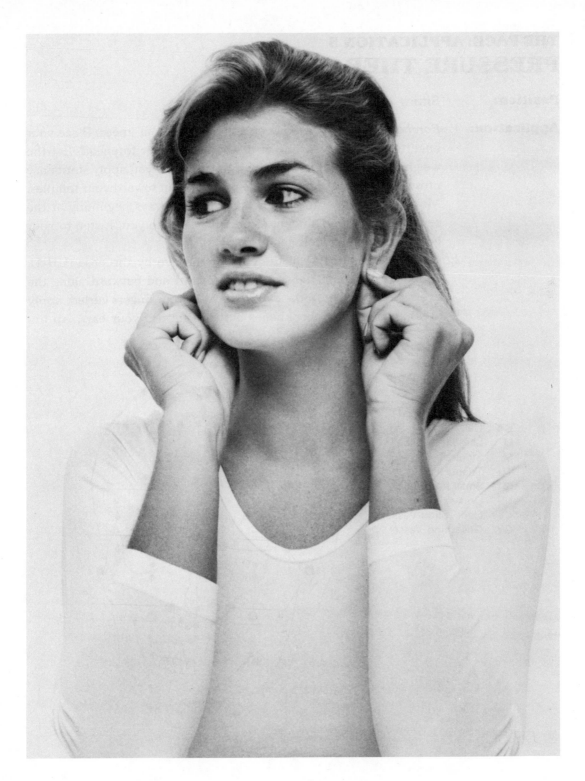

THE FACE: APPLICATION 5
PRESSURE THERAPY

Position: Sitting, using 2 to 4 fingers of each hand.

Application: 1. *Forehead.* Rest your elbows on a table or on your knees. Place your fingertips on your hairline at the center of your forehead. Let the weight of your head fall into your fingertips as you apply stationary pressure. Release and repeat, as you work out toward your temples. Move across the entire forehead in rows, always beginning at the center. Timing and amount of pressure is up to you. Listen to your body and do what feels good.

2. *Eye Sockets.* Starting at the edge of the eye by the nose (UB-1), apply pressure and release. Work upward and outward along the eye socket, just below the eyebrow. With your fingers curled, apply pressure along the cheekbones outward toward your ears. An im-

GB Gall Bladder
LI Large Intestines
St Stomach
TH Triple Heater
SI Small Intestines
UB Urinary Bladder
CV Conception Vessel
GV Governing Vessel

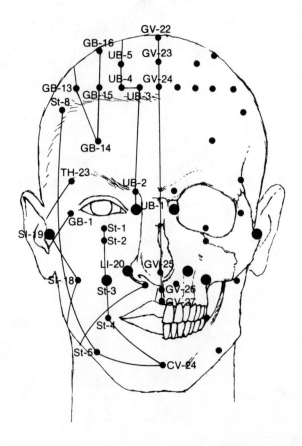

portant point is directly below your pupils (ST-3). Avoid pulling or stretching the eye tissue.

3. *Nostrils.* Starting at the center of your face beside your nostrils (LI-20), apply pressure and release, moving out toward your ears (specifically the tragus). Apply pressure to the tragus point (SI-19).

4. *Upper Lip.* Apply pressure beneath the nose at the center of the upper lip. Work along the upper lip, fingers starting at the center and working outward. Continue down along the outside corners of the mouth and to the jaw. (As though you were following a long mustache.)

5. *Chin.* Starting at the bottom center of the chin, apply pressure and work outward along the jawbone toward the tragus. Apply pressure underneath the jaw along the border with your thumbs.

Beneficial Effects: Helps clear sinus congestion and relieves headaches. Good for hearing, facial beauty, and tired eyes.

Relaxes facial tension and improves circulation.

Major Points:

UB-1	Urinary Bladder
ST-3	Stomach
LI-20	Large Intestine
SI-19	Small Intestine

THE HEAD: APPLICATION 6
SLAPPING

Position: Any, using two hands, four fingers each hand.

Application: 1. Keep fingers together for a harder slap and apart for a lighter slap.
2. Starting at the top of the head, back of neck, or shoulders—slap yourself lightly, gently, lovingly. Continue down arms, chest, legs —all over.
3. This feels wonderful in the shower—great on those mornings when you just can't get up. The shower pressure and water will give you an additional lift.

**Helpful
Hints:**   Do not do so hard as to bruise.
This should not be done on organs or glands.

**Beneficial
Effects:**   Gives a wonderful tingling feeling.
Stimulates circulation to all body systems.

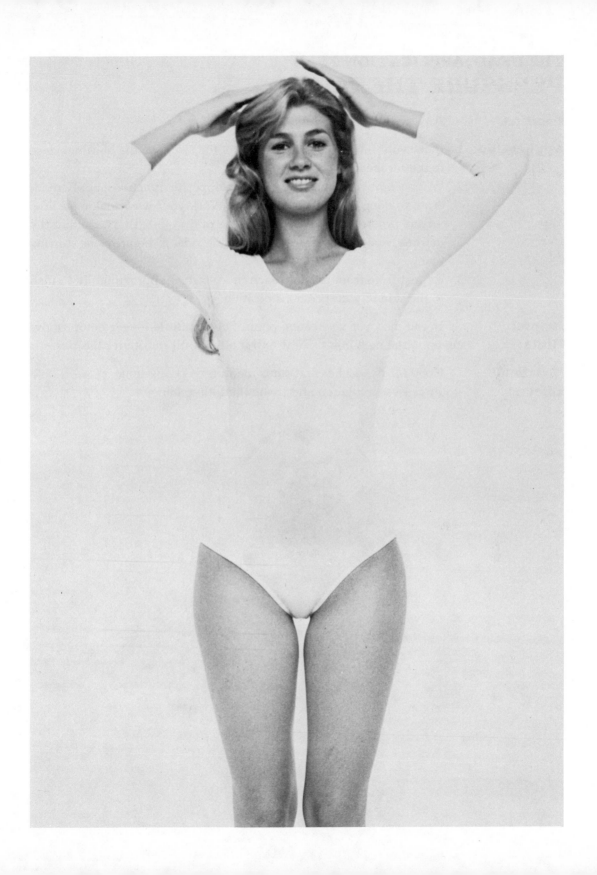

PRESSURE THERAPY

Position: Any, with curled fingers.

Application:
1. Place your fingertips at the center of the scalp, on the hairline, close to the forehead.
2. While slightly pulling your hands in opposite directions, apply moderate to deep amounts of pressure. Work your way, making a line, up and around your head to the base of the skull. Start again at the hairline, about ¼ inch to ½ inch to the side of the previous starting point.
3. Repeat from front to back, each time starting approximately ¼ inch to the side of your previous position.

Helpful Hints: If you discover a sensitive point, hold it a little longer before moving on to the next point. Return to it often until sensitivity has passed.

Beneficial Effects: Good for headaches and sinus membrane congestion. Increases circulation and tissue fluid interchange.

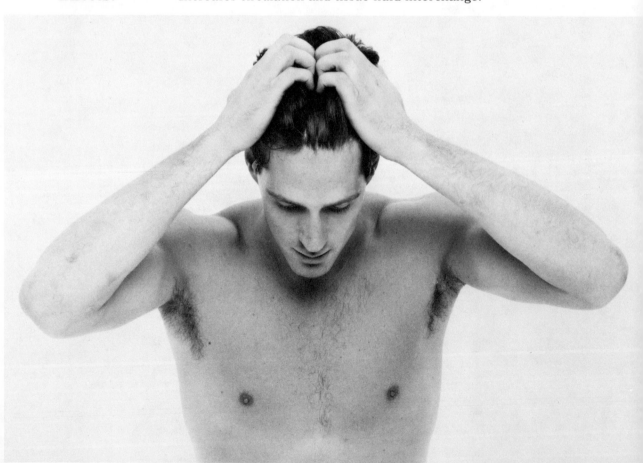

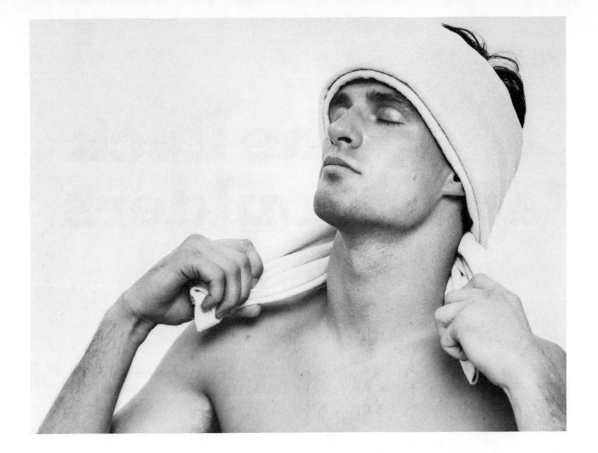

THE HEAD: APPLICATION 8
THE TOWEL VISE

Position: Sitting with hands holding towel.

Application: 1. Fold towel lengthwise three times.
2. Drape center of towel across the forehead.
3. Bring the towel ends to the back of the neck and cross over at the base of the cranium.
4. Bring towel ends forward again.
5. Pulling tightly, but comfortably, use towel like a vise.
6. Exhaling to the count of 5, drop head back, continuing to pull the ends of the towel forward.

Beneficial Effects: A good way to relieve headaches caused by sinus membrane congestion.
Stimulates circulation.

The Neck and Shoulders

NECK STRETCHES

Neck stretches are recommended before and after any self-massage you perform on the neck and shoulder area, or they can be done alone. They are helpful in alleviating neck tension and stretching out neck muscles. *Remember to keep shoulders stationary at all times and to move the head only. Go slowly.*

Application:
1. Bring chin to right shoulder.
2. Bring chin to left shoulder.
3. Drop head back—chin up.
4. Right ear to right shoulder, slowly stretch back.
5. Drop head forward—chin to chest.
6. Left ear to left shoulder, slowly stretch back.
7. Bring head back to center.
8. Repeat, beginning with chin to left shoulder.

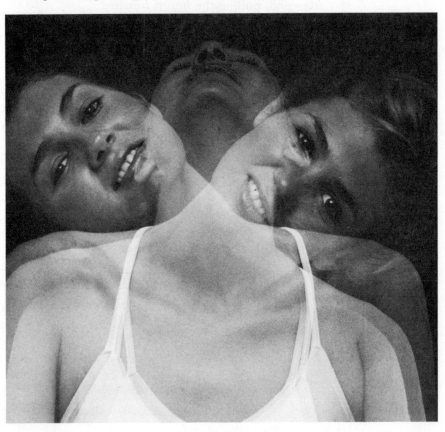

NECK AND SHOULDERS: APPLICATION 2
STROKING

Position: Any, using one or two hands.

Application: 1. Begin just under the head on either side of the spinal column. Keeping four fingers straight, pressure is applied through balls of fingertips. Elbows are pointing up.
2. Stroke forward with pressure going deep into the muscle.
3. Upon exhalation let the *head fall back* into the fingers as the elbows descend, pulling the *hands forward*.
4. With a gliding motion, separate individual muscle fibers.
5. Travel the length of the back side of the neck and outward along the superior border of the shoulder blade.
6. This can be done with both hands simultaneously on both sides.

Helpful Hints: The work is in the upper portions of the fingers, keeping arms and shoulders relaxed.

Apply movement over clothes to avoid burning or apply oil to skin first.

Follow slow breathing patterns.

If you are "nervous," stroke slowly for a more calming effect.

If you are "tired," stroke vigorously for a stimulating effect.

Beneficial Effects: Relieves excessive muscular tension.

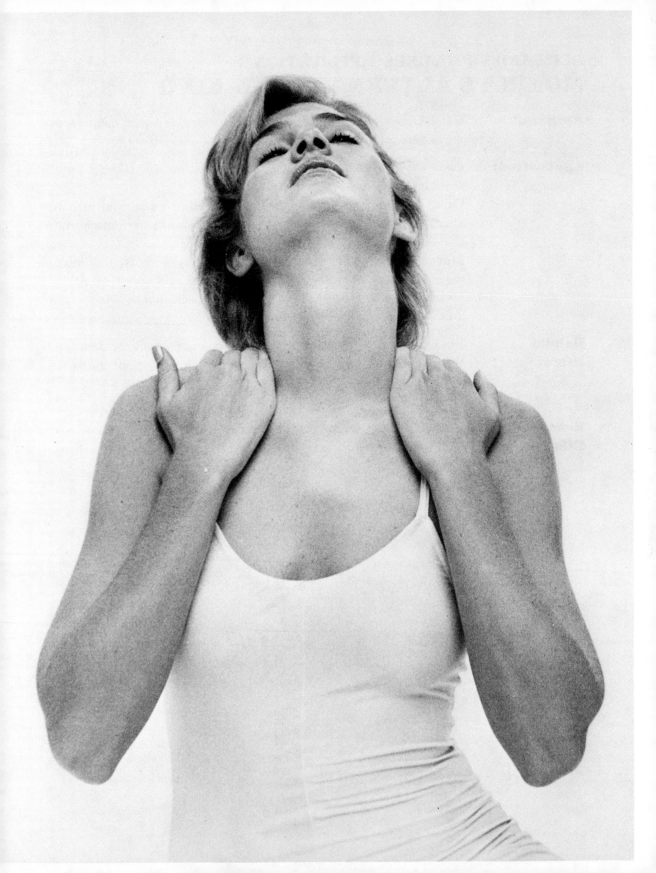

MONIKA'S ALTERNATING RAKING

Position: Can be done standing, sitting, or lying; using one or two hands, four strong fingers with each.

Application:
1. Place hands on either side of shoulder muscles, superior border of shoulder blade, or trapezius muscle.
2. Using the palms as an anchor or support, fingers are put into an alternating walking motion as they slightly pinch the muscle into the palm.
3. Movement of fingers does not have to be synchronized or alternated in any order, and should be slow, deep, and unrestrained.
4. Head is either dropped forward or tilted back slightly so that the muscle is more accessible.

Helpful Hints: For extra leverage you can rest your elbows on a table or desk.

Stop when your fingers get tired. Avoid working a specific area for more than 5 minutes.

Remember to relax and follow normal breathing patterns.

Beneficial Effects: Passively stretches and warms muscles.

This is excellent for treating localized tension in the neck and shoulder areas.

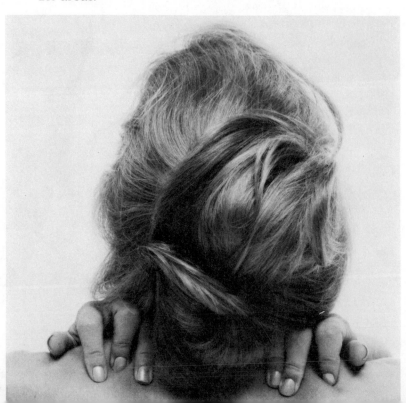

NECK AND SHOULDERS: APPLICATION 4

VIBRATION

Position: Sitting or lying; using one hand, three fingers.

Application: 1. Take one hand across chest and place three middle fingers on the neck to the side of the spinal column.

2. Hand should be slightly cupped and contact should be made with the balls of the fingertips.

3. Without breaking contact on the skin's surface apply pressure and shake fingers back and forth vigorously for 3 seconds.

4. Release and move down to the next vertebrae. Repeat. Continue down the back of the neck and along the superior border of the shoulder blade.

5. Reach down the spinal column as far as you comfortably can by raising your elbow.

6. Repeat entire procedure on opposite side.

Helpful Hints: If the muscle is too tight, drop your ear slightly to the side you are working, or try it lying down.

Stop and shake out hands if they become tired or strained.

Beneficial Effects: Aids in dispersing metabolic waste products.

Relieves excessive muscular tension.

NECK AND SHOULDERS: APPLICATION 5
THE PINCH . . . one good pinch deserves another!

Position: Sitting with head slightly tilted back or, better, lying on your back. Using one hand with palm for support or using thumb and opposing middle and index fingers of both hands, alternating rhythmically. Back and neck muscles must be in a relaxed posture.

Application: *Soft pinch*

1. Straddling the spine with palm and four fingers opposing, pick up the muscle at the back of the neck, allowing your head to fall freely into the movement.
2. Pinch it lightly while gently pulling it away from the bone.
3. Release gradually, allowing the fingers to glide off the muscle.
4. Continue down the back of the neck and along the shoulder muscle. Treating shoulder muscles is best done with one hand crossing chest to the opposite shoulder. It is better to work on a relaxed muscle.

Variation: *For a harder pinch*

1. Perform the same pinching movement but this time only using the thumb, index, and middle fingers.
2. Index and middle fingers will be opposing thumb while straddling spine.
3. Alternate hands as you work down the neck and across the shoulders.

Helpful Hints: This application is the most effective when done lying down. Recommended time for treatment is one minute per side.

Beneficial Effects: Stretches muscle fibers. Stimulates circulation and lymphatic drainage.

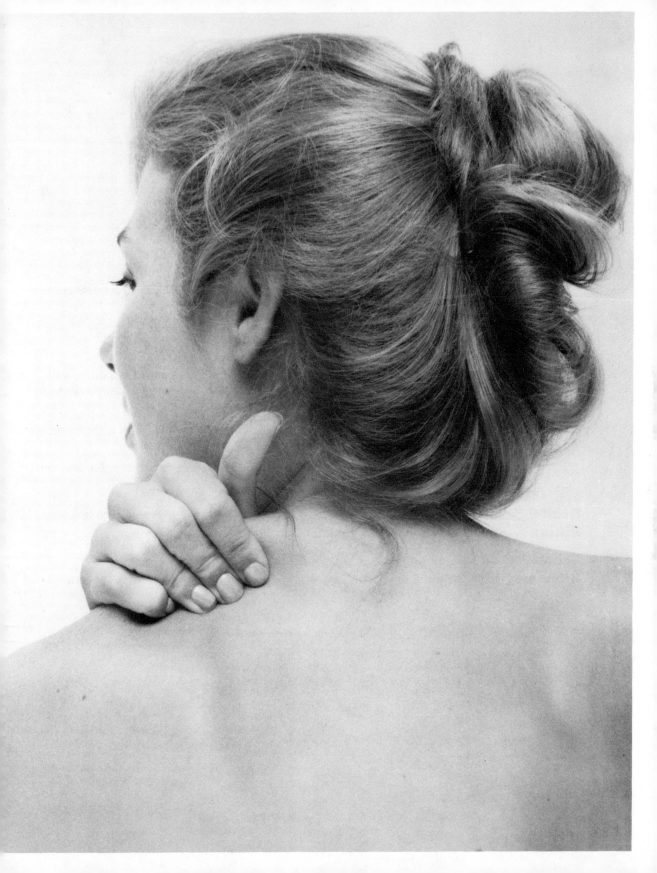

NECK AND SHOULDERS: APPLICATION 6
PUSH-ROLLING

Position: Sitting or lying down.

Using both hands, three strongest fingers in each hand.

Head is relaxed and should be allowed to fall freely back into fingers.

Application: 1. Starting at the base of the cranium, place one hand on each side of the spinal column.

2. Using the three strongest fingers in each hand (index, middle, and fourth), push one side and then the other toward the center of the spinal column.

3. With minimum but deep pressure, alternate hands with a rhythmic motion down the spine.

4. Proceed down the neck as far as you can go comfortably. Repeat 5 times.

Helpful Hints: Remember to stay relaxed and allow head to fall freely into fingers. When you feel tension in your hands it is time to stop.

Beneficial Effects: Aids in the relief of excessive muscular tension.

Stimulates circulation and indirectly improves muscle contractibility.

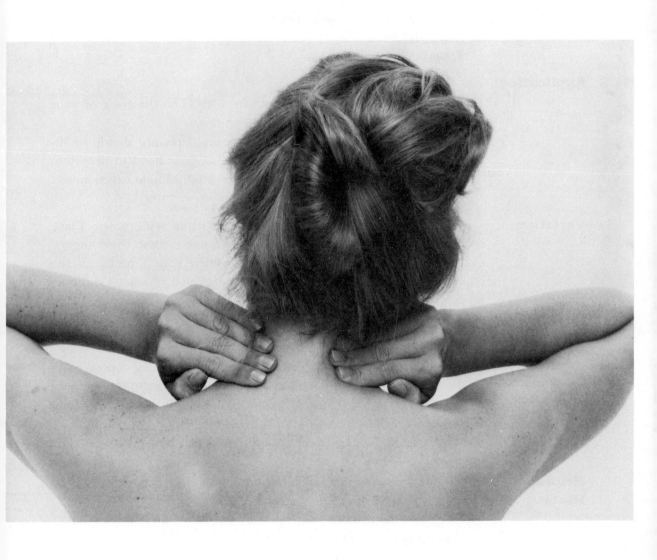

PRESSURE THERAPY

Position:　　　Sitting or lying on your back.

Use your thumbs on your neck and your index and middle fingers on your shoulders.

Treat bilaterally.

Application: *The Neck*

1. Position your thumb at the base of the skull on the back of your neck on the occipital border (GB-20 points).

2. Upon exhalation apply *stationary pressure*. Pressure should be directed up and into the head. By allowing your head to drop into your thumb the necessary pressure is created. Muscle exertion isn't needed. Inhale as you release.

Variation:　　　Try applying pressure to GB-20 points while lying down. Place both of your hands on the base of your head so that your fingers, overlapping, are cradling your head. Position your thumbs on the points. Exhale and apply pressure. Inhale as you release. Continue, moving your hands and thumbing your way down either side of the neck along the column.

Application: *The Shoulders*

The points on the shoulders are best affected by bringing one hand across the chest to the opposite shoulder. With a clawed hand, apply deep *stationary pressure*, using the index and middle fingers. Pressure is applied along the shoulder toward the arm joint. The points to be affected are GB-21 and LI-15. These points can be held longer than the points on the neck.

Helpful Hints:　　　Recommended timing: exhale and hold for a count of 5; inhale and release for a count of 3.

Help shoulder muscles stay relaxed by focusing on your breathing. Specific points can be held 10 to 15 seconds 3 times.

Beneficial Effects:　　　Improves circulation.

Aids in the relief of stiffness in neck and shoulder joints, headaches, and shoulder tension.

Major Points:　　　GB-20; 21　　Gall Bladder

LI-15　　　　Large Intestine

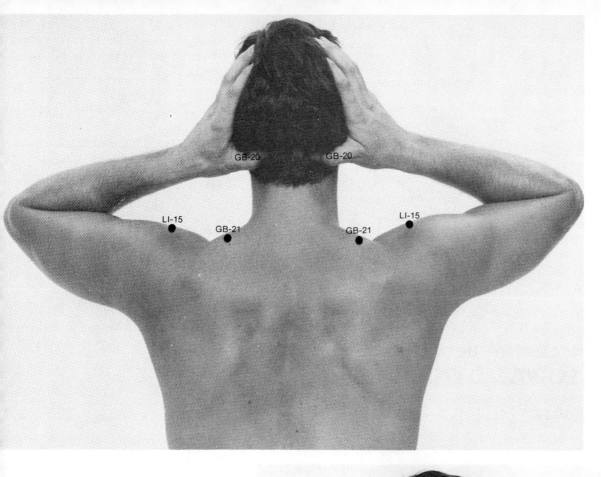

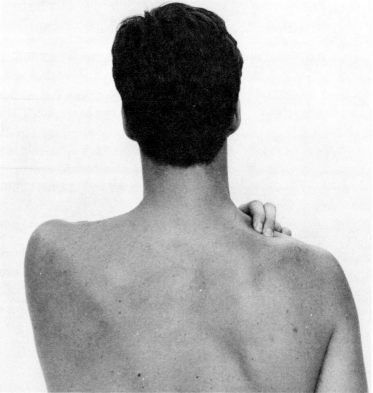

Towel Dynamics

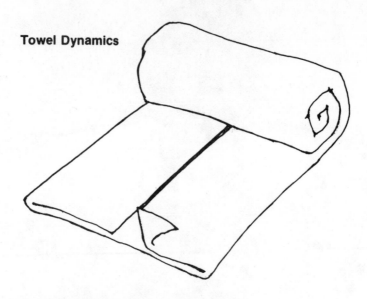

NECK AND SHOULDERS: APPLICATION 8
TOWEL DYNAMICS

Exercise 1:   *The Spinal*

(Applied on cervical curve [base of cranium] and lumbar [small of back] anterior curves)

Position: Lying on your back on a flat surface.

Application: 1. Fold a towel lengthwise so that the sides meet at the center. (It will look like closed window shutters). Now roll the towel up tightly.
2. While lying down on a flat surface place this tightly rolled towel in the cervical curve of the neck at the base of the head.
3. Remain in this position for 15–20 minutes. You can experiment by rolling the rolled towel up and down your neck and back.
4. This should also be applied to the lumbar curve (the small of the back). Place the rolled towel under your back and repeat the above steps.

Beneficial Effects: Opens up neck and lower back anterior vertebral articulation (natural curve of the spine), as it bilaterally sets the tissue fluid balance, thereby reducing pain caused by excessive amounts of tension.

This is excellent for reducing neck and shoulder tension. Apply 15 minutes before bedtime, to prevent early morning stiffness.

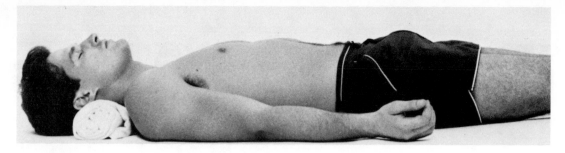

Exercise 2: *The Roll*

Position: Sitting with hands holding towel.

Application: 1. Fold towel lengthwise into thirds.
2. Holding towel ends, position your head in the center of the towel around the base of the cranium.
3. While supporting head with towel, allow head to fall freely back into towel. (As though the towel were a sling for your head.)
4. Pull one side of the towel and then the other. Pull back and forth, rotating the cranium.
5. Follow normal breathing patterns and let the towel do the work.

Beneficial Effects: Stimulates mobility in the cervical vertebrae.

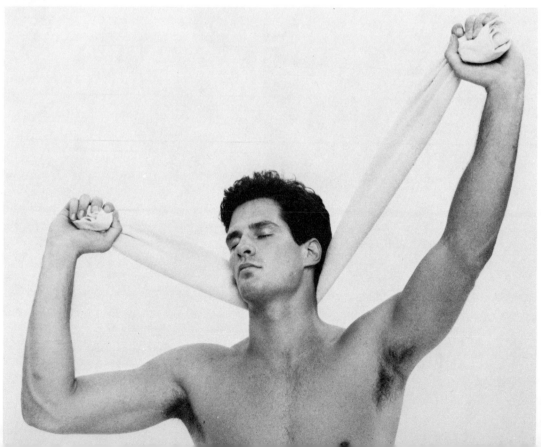

Hands and Arms

SIMPLE HAND STRETCH

Position: Any

Application: *Fingers*

1. Interlock fingers.
2. As you stretch your arms out, invert your fingers and hold.
3. Stretch to the left and hold.
4. Stretch to the right and hold.

Wrist

1. Tightly lock your fingers around the wrist of the receiving hand (like a bracelet).
2. Circle your hand to the right, bending at the wrist, 3 to 5 times, while supporting the ligaments.
3. Then rotate 3 to 5 times to the left.
4. Repeat on the opposite hand.

Beneficial Effects: Quick relief for tired, tense hands.

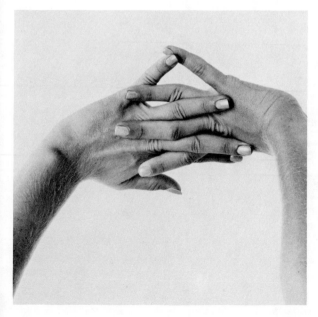
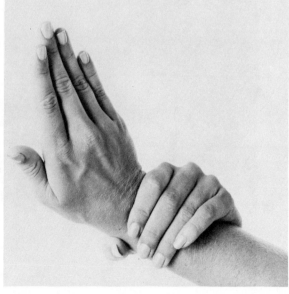

HANDS: APPLICATION 2
STROKING

Position: Any that is comfortable. The work is done with the hands.

Application:
1. With the ball of the thumb of the giving hand, begin stroking the receiving hand at the base of the palm and work toward the fingers.
2. Stroke back and forth with deep, concentrated strokes.
3. Stroke down each finger and on each joint space. Stroke the sides of the fingers one by one.
4. Flip the receiving hand over and stroke down and in between each finger.
5. Reverse roles, stroking opposite hand.

Beneficial Effects: Improves circulation and relieves tension and fatigue in the hands.

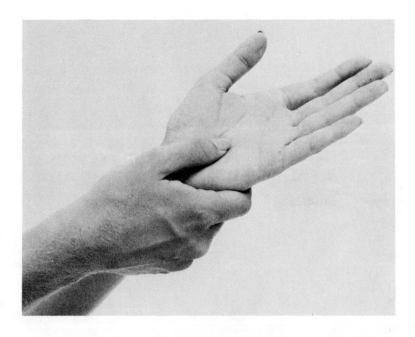

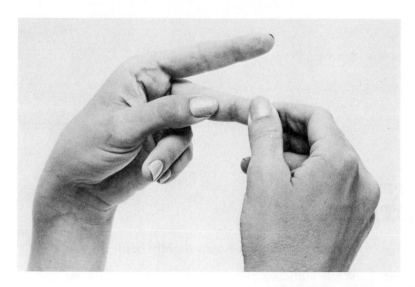

JOINT ROTATION

Position: Any, with one hand giving and one hand receiving. Use your thumb and index finger.

Application:
1. Each finger has three joints that can be rotated sideways. The thumb has only two.
2. With the thumb and index finger of the giving hand, hold firmly between the joint spaces of the fingers of the receiving hand. You will be holding and rotating one joint at a time.
3. While holding one joint space, simply twist the joint space sideways to the left and then to the right 3 to 4 times. Move on to the next joint space and repeat.
4. After you have rotated each joint go on to the next finger. Do all of your fingers and both thumbs.

Helpful Hints: Stabilizing the joint being rotated provides a more effective rotation. This is done with the thumb of the hand that's being affected. Place the thumb on the side of the finger just below the joint. By doing this only the individual joint will be rotated. *Simply, you stabilize below the joint while you rotate above it.*

Beneficial Effects: Helps maintain joint mobility.
Helps relieve tired, stiff hands.

ARMS: APPLICATION 4
ARM STRETCHES

Position: Standing with your knees slightly bent.

Application:
1. While standing place your feet about 12 inches apart and interlock your thumbs behind your back.
2. As you inhale deeply, bend backward as far as comfort and balance allow, pulling your arms out from your body.
3. As you exhale slowly, come forward and bend over as you bring your arms up over your back as far as possible.
4. Hold the position. Upon exhalation, push the position a little further.
5. Inhale, slowly straightening up to your original position.
6. Reverse the interlocking thumbs and repeat the entire stretch.

Beneficial Effects:
Stretches out the Lung meridian and the Large Intestine meridian as it stretches out the arm muscles.

This stretch is also very soothing to the middle back.

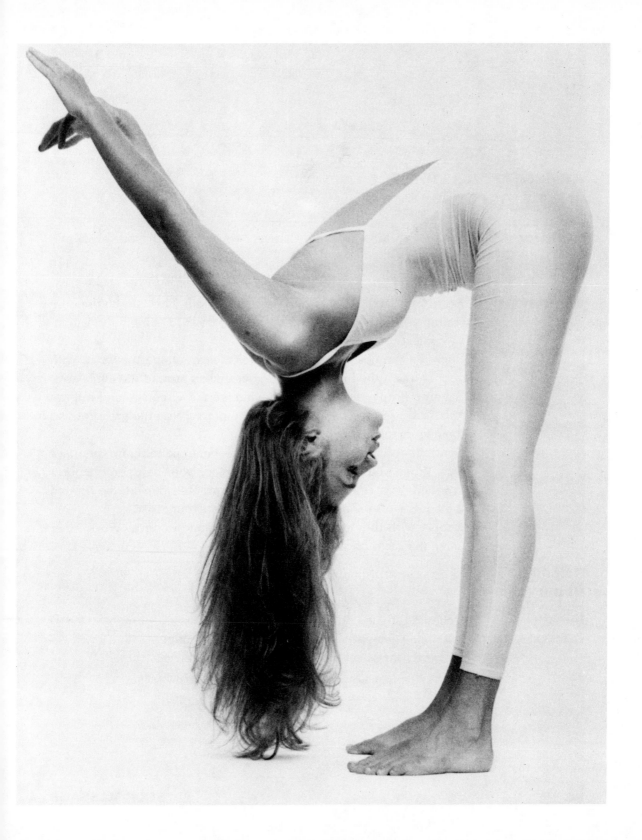

ARMS: APPLICATION 5
ROLLING

Position: Any comfortable position that lets you work with your arms and hands.

Use your palm or thumb with opposing four fingers.

Application:
1. Begin by relaxing the muscle being affected. This can be done by resting your arm in your lap or, if lying down, resting your arm on your chest.
2. Begin on the fleshier portion of the forearm above the wrist, with your palm on the inner arm and your fingers around the outer arm.
3. Squeeze firmly, as though your hand were a vise grip, and roll the muscle around the bone. Allow the palm to create the pressure and the fingers to stabilize the movement.
4. Continue rolling the muscle around the bone, palming up the inner arm. When you reach your shoulder, place your palm on the outer arm and your fingers on your inner arm. Roll the muscle around the bone, working down your outer arm to your wrist.
5. Repeat with the opposite hand on your opposite arm. Work inner and outer arms once.

Helpful Hints: Keep your arms and shoulders relaxed.

Beneficial Effects: Relieves fatigue in arms.

Maintains circulation and tissue fluid interchange.

Indirectly increases the muscles' ability to contract.

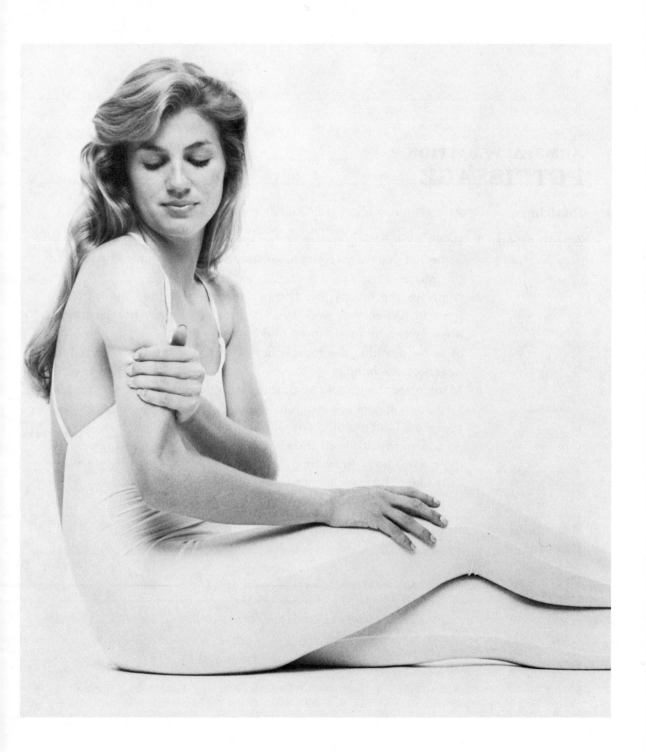

ARMS: APPLICATION 6
PETRISSAGE

Position: Any, with one hand giving while the opposite arm receives.

Application: 1. Begin by applying petrissage on any of the fleshier parts (muscle bodies) of your arm. Remember that this is a rhythmic kneading of the muscle.

2. Apply to the biceps and triceps muscles, and then apply to the forearm. When you work the forearm, or smaller muscle groups, use only two to three fingers and opposing thumb.

3. Start by pinching the muscle lightly between the thumb and four fingers of one hand.

4. Manipulate the muscle by pushing with your thumb while you pull your four fingers toward your palm, continually twisting, gliding, squeezing, and molding your fingers around the tissue.

5. As you push with your thumb and pull with your four fingers, roll the muscle body, traveling the full length of the arm. Glide vertically along the muscle body without breaking contact.

6. Repeat on the opposite arm using the opposite hand.

Beneficial Effects: Increases circulation and lymphatic drainage.

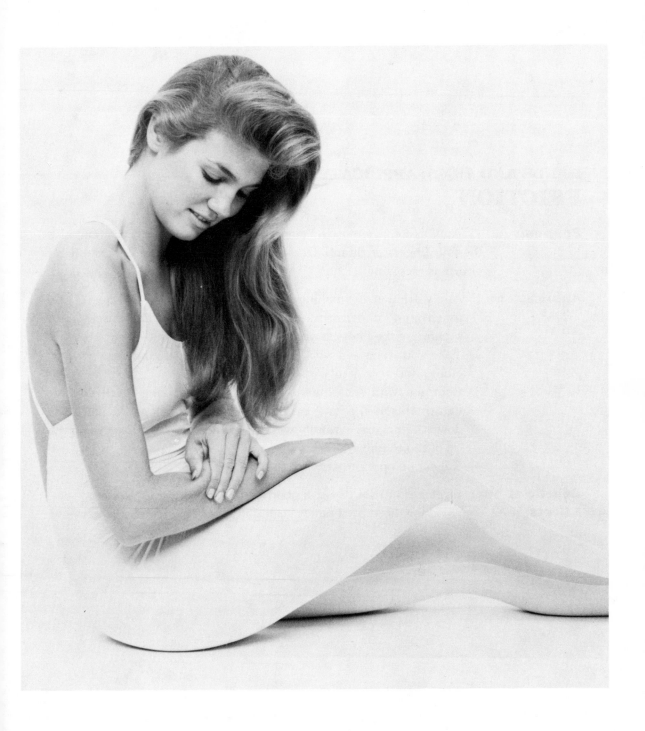

HANDS AND ARMS: APPLICATION 7
FRICTION

Position: Any, as long as muscle being affected is in a relaxed position. Use the four fingers or thumb. One hand is giving while the opposite hand or arm is receiving.

Application: 1. Apply friction by making small circles along the muscles of the forearm and upper arm. Travel with the grain of the muscle fiber, separating the fibers as you work the inner and outer arm.
2. Take your time and work slowly, but deeply, around the shoulder, elbow, and wrist joints.
3. Continue with the thumb or four fingers making small circular movements on the inner and outer hand. Glide along the palm and down the fingers, carefully working individual joint spaces with the tip of the thumb.
4. Repeat on opposite arm and hand.

Beneficial Effects: Stretches muscle tissue, limbering up joints.
Good for those tired hands, especially for writers and secretaries.

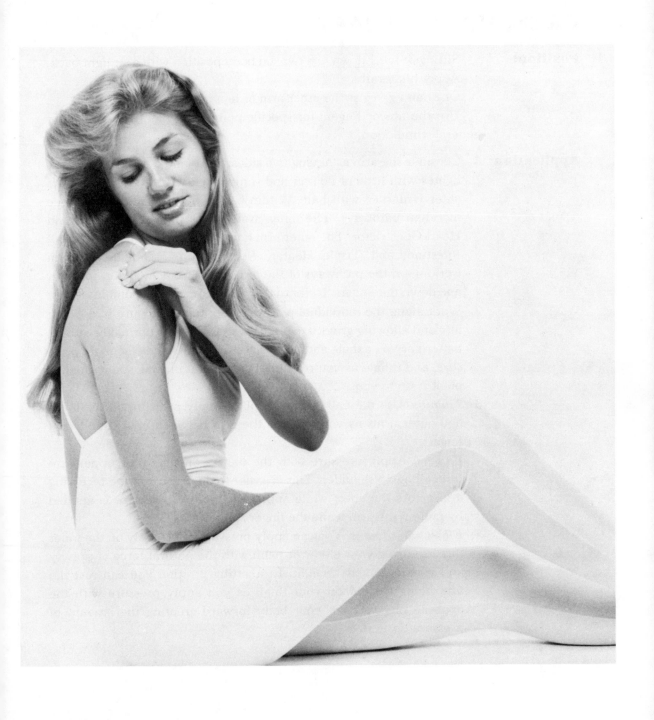

PRESSURE THERAPY

Position: Sitting or lying down in a relaxed body position with a straight back. Apply bilaterally.

One hand gives as the other arm or hand receives.

Use thumbs or fingers for specific points and palms or elbows for general stimulation.

Application: 1. Consider the arm as having two sides: inner and outer. The inner is lighter with little or no hair and is more sensitive to the touch. The outer is darker with hair. Within each side of the arm are three meridian pathways. The inner arm houses the Lung, Heart, and Heart Constrictor. The outer arm houses the Large Intestine, Small Intestine, and Triple Heater. *Recommended Direction:* When working on the pathways of the arm, work from shoulder, to wrist, and down the fingers. Refer to the charts for specific point locations.

2. Work along the individual pathways, applying pressure by leaning into and allowing gravity to do the work. Follow a normal breathing pattern as you exhale and apply deep, concentrated *stationary pressure,* and inhale as you release. The amount of time spent on each point is up to you.

3. *Thumbs.* Use the ball of the thumb to apply pressure on the inner and outer arms as you squeeze the arm between your thumb and fingers.

4. *Fingers.* Apply pressure with the fingers on the outer upper arm from elbow to shoulder. This is easier to do if you rest the receiving arm across the chest while applying pressure. Pressure is applied by pulling the arm while the fingers penetrate.

5. *Elbows and Palms.* You can apply pressure effortlessly on the inner forearm using your elbow or palm with the natural force of gravity and your own body weight. In a sitting position you can rest the arm being treated on your thigh as you apply pressure with the opposite elbow. Lean your body forward creating the amount of pressure desired.

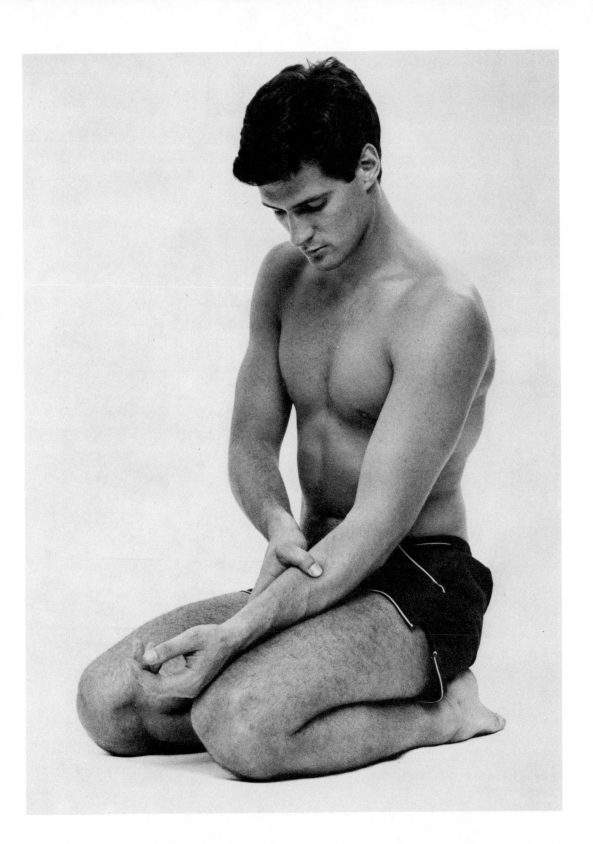

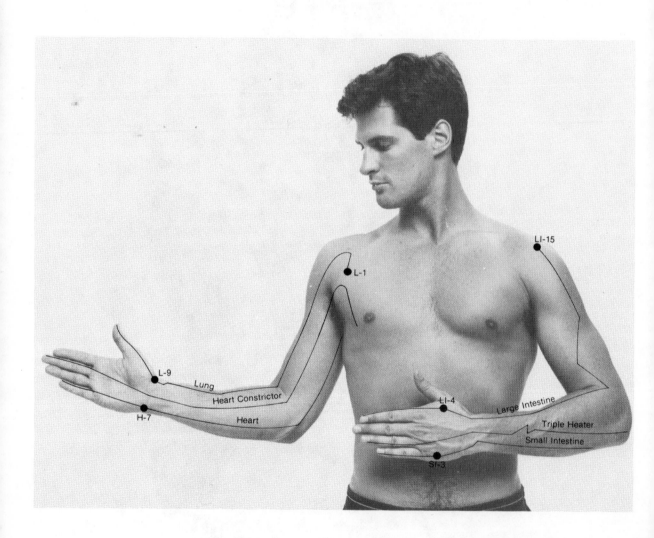

**Helpful
Hints:**   Feel for the individual points. They will be more sensitive to the touch.

Take time with your body, keeping your shoulders relaxed as you work with your breath.

Avoid applying on the site of pain—work above and below it.

Specific points can be held 10 to 15 seconds and done 3 times. Hold any sensitive points longer until a pulse is felt.

**Beneficial
Effects:**   Improves circulation and helps to maintain good health.

Good for numbness in fingers, insomnia, arm spasms and weariness in the arms, and headaches.

**Major
Points:**   H-7   Heart
SI-3   Small Intestine
L-1-9   Lung
LI-4-15   Large Intestine

Chest and Abdominal Region

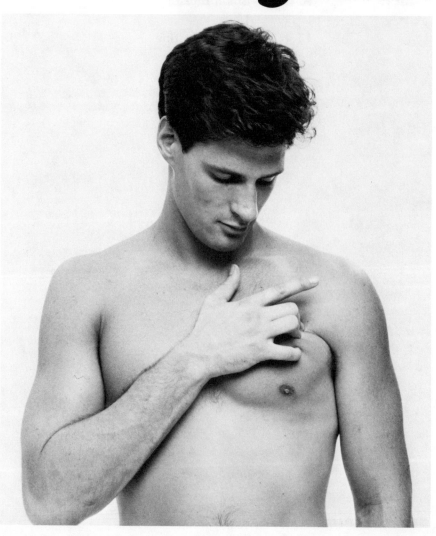

STROKING

Position: Lying on your back, or sitting. Using four fingertips of one hand.

Application:
1. This is a firm stroking movement done with varying amounts of pressure.
2. Begin by the shoulder joint, stroking inward below the collarbone and above the breasts. Stroke toward the center of your breastbone.
3. Stroke down the breastbone (sternum).
4. Then stretch out the muscles by raising one hand and resting it over your head. Stroke along the opposite rib cage, molding your fingers to your ribs as you move your hand in between and along the bones. Work along your ribs toward your side, going as far as comfort allows.
5. Change hands for opposite sides and repeat. Recommended time: 5 minutes per side.

Variation: Using Monika's Alternate Finger Raking:

1. Apply around the insertion tendon of the pectoral muscle. This is by the shoulder joint. Anchor your palm for leverage near the top center of the breastbone. Stroke by alternating your fingers and pulling them in toward your palm.
2. As you stroke with alternating fingers, draw your shoulder back, stretching out the muscles being affected.

Helpful Hints: This is a very relaxing, easy movement to do. Try to do some deep breathing while you stroke.

Whenever your fingers get tired, shake them out and continue from where you stopped.

Beneficial Effects: Increases circulation and lymphatic drainage.

Soothes and relaxes fatigued muscles.

Helps slumped, tired shoulders by releasing and stretching out the muscles.

CHEST: APPLICATION 2
FRICTION

Position:

Lying on your back with your knees bent, or sitting.

Using the balls of the fingertips.

It is easiest to use your right hand when working on your left side, and your left hand when working on your right side.

Applications:

1. Keep your shoulders relaxed, and follow normal breathing patterns. Make small circular movements with the balls of your fingertips as you travel, separating the muscle fibers.
2. Work around the shoulder joint where the arm and shoulder meet.
3. Work along the collarbone above the breasts, down the breastbone (sternum) between the breasts, and then along the ribs under the breasts.
4. If you are lying down you can stretch out the muscles along the ribs by resting your free hand above your head.
5. Change hands and massage opposite side.
6. Recommended time: up to 5 minutes for each side.

Helpful Hints:

Now is a good time for women to do their breast self-examination by making light gliding circular movements around the breast. Starting on the outside borders, working toward the nipple, explore and feel for lumps that were not there during your last self-examination.

Beneficial Effects:

Maintains range of motion when applying friction movements around the shoulder joint.

Stimulates circulation and tissue fluid interchange.

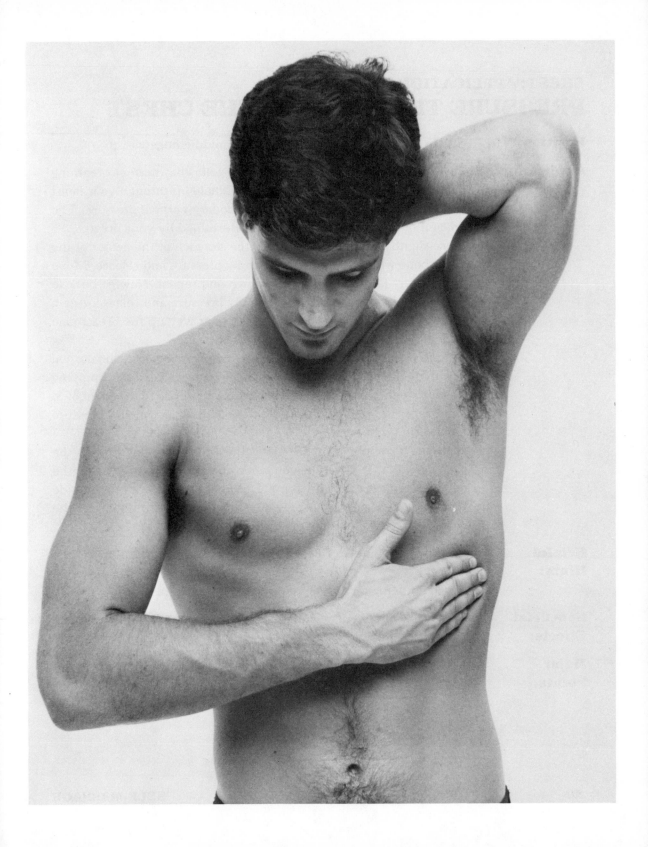

CHEST: APPLICATION 3
PRESSURE THERAPY FOR THE CHEST

Position: Sitting or lying down, using index and middle fingers.

Application:
1. Focus on your breath as your center, following normal breathing patterns. Inhale down to your navel. Exhale up through your heart and into your hands as you apply *stationary vertical pressure*. The amount of pressure applied will be determined by your breath.
2. Place slightly curled fingers above the stomach at the center of the breastbone where the ribs meet. Apply pressure and release. Move your fingers laterally out ¼ of an inch and repeat. Now go back to the center, but up ¼ of an inch. Apply pressure and release. Again go out ¼ of an inch and repeat. Work your way up the breastbone until you reach the collarbone in rows of two.
3. Timing is individual. You can hold a point, following your normal breathing pattern (slowed down a bit, of course), or exhale, applying pressure to the count of 5 and release as you inhale to the count of 3. Hold sensitive points longer. You can lighten up on the pressure and wait for a pulse.
4. Continue to apply pressure along the collarbone out toward the shoulder joint. It is best if you work one side at a time, using the opposite hand to apply pressure. This keeps the muscles on the side being affected relaxed. Apply pressure in two rows beneath the collarbone. Repeat on the opposite side.

Helpful Hints: Keep your shoulders relaxed, as the work is done with your wrist and fingers.

Avoid applying any pressure directly on the glands.

Beneficial Effects: Beneficial in relieving symptoms due to cold, coughs, and asthma. Improves circulation and helps to maintain good health.

Major Points: L-1   Lung

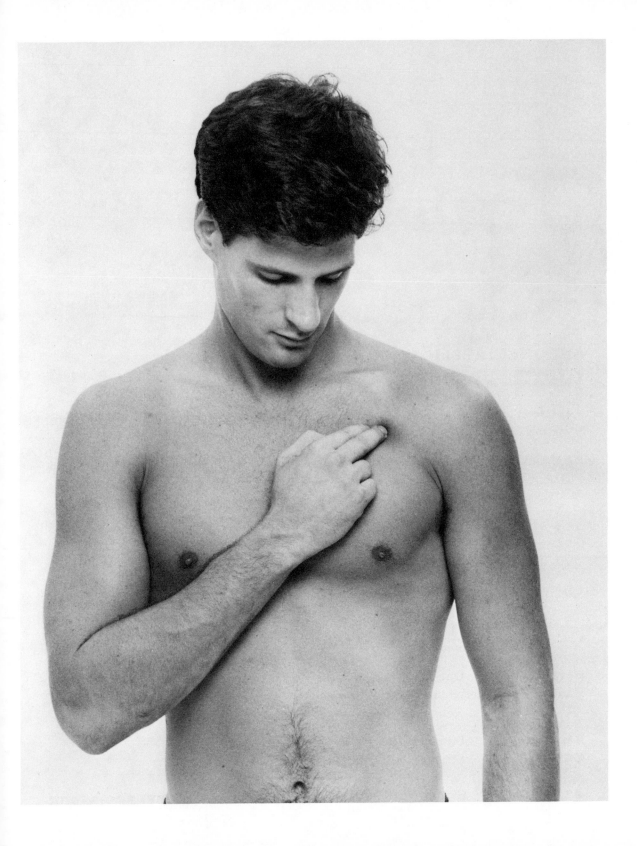

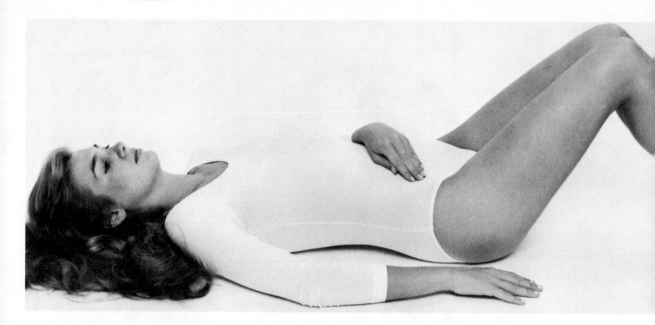

ABDOMEN: APPLICATION 4
CIRCLES

Position: Lying on your back with your knees bent, using the balls of four fingertips.

Application: 1. When performing this movement your fingers will make small, deep circles as they travel clockwise along the bony borders around the abdomen. This should be a circular, sliding motion performed without breaking contact with the skin's surface.
2. With your left hand, begin along the lower right hipbone. Slowly, make small circles as you travel up the abdominal wall following the large intestine. Proceed horizontally under the rib cage.
3. When you reach the center below the diaphragm you can change hands so that you are using your right hand as you work across the left side and down the left abdominal border to the lower left hipbone.

Helpful Hints: One hand can be placed on the other for more strength. Follow normal breathing patterns.
Remember to keep your shoulders relaxed.

Beneficial Effects: Stimulates peristaltic response.
Stretches and strengthens abdominal muscles.

SELF-MASSAGE

VIBRATION

Position: Lying on your back with knees bent, using the balls of four finger-tips.

Application:
1. Vibration will be done along the large intestine, starting by the lower right hip.
2. This is a simple vibration movement that will jiggle the large intestine as you move up the right side of the abdomen, going left horizontally under the rib cage, and down the left side of the abdomen to the lower left hipbone.
3. The movement comes from the wrist and four fingers as you apply pressure and shake the fingers back and forth without breaking contact with the skin's surface.
4. Recommended time: vibrate for 3 seconds and release as you move along the intestine.

Variation: A flat hand can be used to apply horizontal vibration above the navel and along the rib cage.

Helpful Hints: Use alternating hands if your hands tire quickly.
Remember to keep your shoulders relaxed, as the movement comes from the wrist and four fingers.

Beneficial Effects: Stimulates peristaltic response.
Stimulates circulation and nerve response in the area.

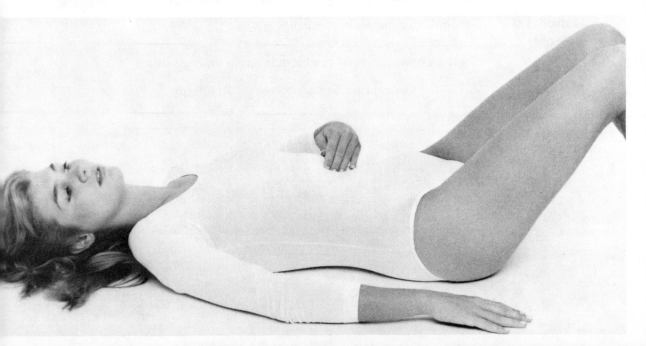

ABDOMEN: APPLICATION 6
PRESSURE THERAPY

Position: Lying on your back with your knees bent, using two hands and four fingers.

Application:

1. Begin by getting in touch with your breathing. Place your hands just below your navel. As you inhale through your nose, bring your breath into your hands. As you exhale through your mouth follow your breath with your eyes and ears. Breathe slowly and deeply 5 to 10 times. Feel yourself relaxing and letting go. Pressure therapy should be applied as you follow these breathing patterns.

2. The angle of pressure is vertical, going into the abdomen, and just to the sides of the bony borders. Beginning just above the pubic bone, you will apply pressure therapy going from right to left as you make a full circle around the abdominal wall.

3. Start by inverting your hands. Your fingers can be back to back or overlapping. Positioning your fingers just above the pubic bone, inhale into your hands. Upon exhalation apply stationary pressure, holding to the count of 5. Release to the count of 3 as you inhale.

4. Synchronize your breath with the pressure application as you continue to the right, going up the right abdominal wall, left horizontally (below the rib cage), down the left abdominal wall, and back to the starting position above the pubic bone.

5. As you travel around the abdomen the hands remain parallel to the bony borders, moving 1 to 1½ inches after each application.

Beneficial Effects:
Stimulates peristaltic response.
Helps alleviate menstrual discomfort.
Helps maintain good health in internal organ systems.

Major Point:
CV-6   Conception Vessel, "ocean of Ki energy"

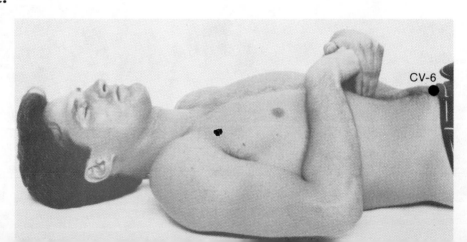

CV-6

The Back

THE BACK: APPLICATION 1
LUMBAR STRETCH

Position: Lying on your back on a flat surface while focusing on your breath.

Application: 1. Upon inhalation bring one knee up toward your chest and leave one leg straight.
2. As you exhale, fold your arms around your knee and draw your head and shoulders in to your knee.
3. Hold this position as you take a few normal breaths.
4. Upon exhalation, release arms and then shoulders and head as you straighten out your knee, ending back in original position.
5. Repeat with opposite leg.
6. Then repeat bringing both legs to your chest simultaneously, hold the position, and release. Your breath and movements should be as one.

Beneficial Effects: Stretches out lower back muscles.
Good for chronic lower back pain, caused by muscular tension.

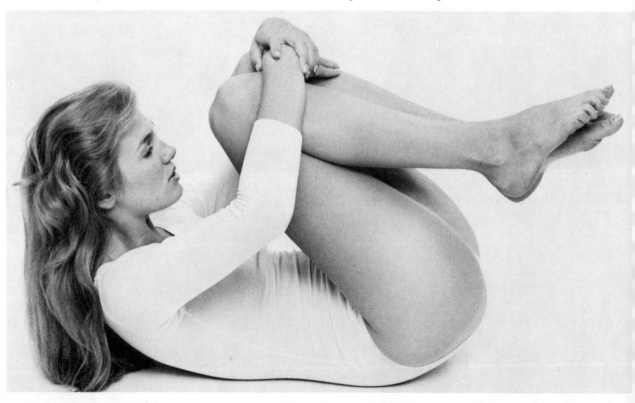

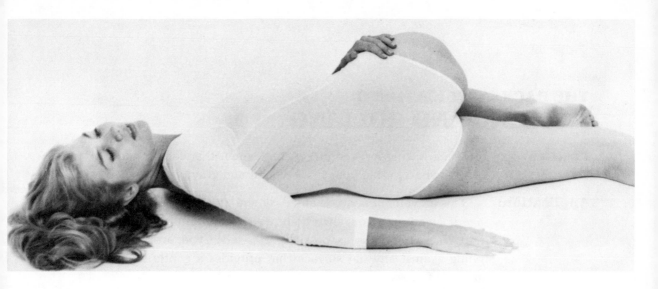

THE BACK: APPLICATION 2
SPINAL TWIST

Position: Lying on your back on the floor with arms resting by your side.

Application:
1. Begin by focusing on your breathing. Let your deep breathing relax and calm you.
2. Upon inhalation, slowly bring your right knee up to your chest.
3. As you exhale, slowly twist your pelvis and drop your knee to the left side of your body, turning head to your right. These movements should be done simultaneously.
4. Hold this position as you breathe slowly and deeply 3 to 4 times.
5. Upon inhalation, bring your knee and head back to the center of your body.
6. As you exhale, lower knee and straighten your leg out, returning to your original position.
7. Repeat, as you breathe deeply, on the opposite side: left knee to your right side while your head is turned to the left. Remember that your knee and head move in opposite directions.

Helpful Hints: Synchronize the movement with your breath.
I recommend this movement daily.

Beneficial Effects: Increases mobility in lumbar and sacral spine.

THE BACK: APPLICATION 3
ROCKING AND ROLLING

Position: Lying, sitting, or standing. A movement that can be done anytime and anywhere, using your body weight and gravity.

Application: This movement is quick and easy and involves no hands. The massage is given with your own body weight and natural movement, and is to be as effortless as possible. Basically, you are rocking and/or rolling against any flat surface that provides a gentle but substantial amount of pressure.

1. *Lying down.* On your back with your knees bent and your feet flat on the surface, wiggle and roll your whole body from side to side and up and down along your spine. Now rock your body up and down along your spine while you clasp your arms around your knees, bringing them toward your chest, rocking and rolling slowly.
2. *Standing against a wall.* Stand with your feet flat and approximately one foot away from a wall. Lean into the wall so that it supports your body weight. Roll back and forth against the wall. Movement is synchronized with your breath.
3. *Sitting in a hard cushioned chair.* Roll your back against the chair horizontally. Experiment by lifting your shoulders up and down, keeping shoulders relaxed as you roll.

Helpful Hints: Try this movement in your car when stuck in traffic, at the office in your desk chair, or against the wall.

Work the back for 5 minutes, keeping your breathing slow and deep.

Beneficial Effects: This is a quick relaxer for tired tense backs.

Stimulates and wakes up your back. Great for "office slouch."

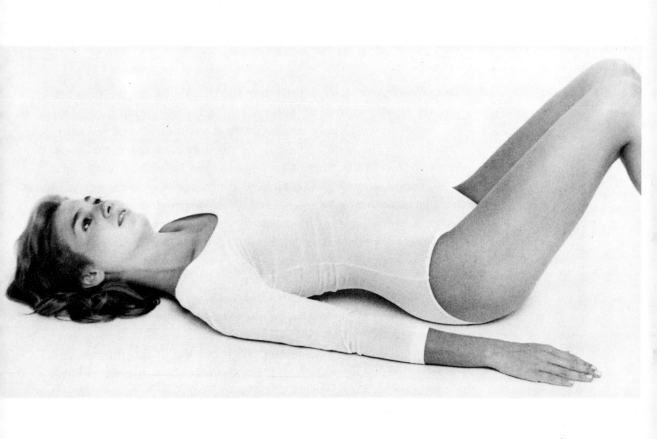

THE BACK: APPLICATION 4
STROKING

Position: Sitting or lying on your side with knees bent, using thumbs, flat of four fingers, knuckles, and back of hand. Be creative!

Posture is to remain relaxed at all times.

Application: With bent elbow(s) and arm(s) reach behind you and up the spinal column as far as comfort allows for each particular movement. Stroking is applied horizontally and vertically on the back with different parts of the hand.

1. *Using the thumb(s).* With the flat of the thumb, for deeper penetration, stroke down along the sides of the spinal column to the coccyx (tail bone) as you apply moderate to deep amounts of pressure. Repeat with the thumb, making vertical strokes down the back. Also stroke with the thumbs by beginning at the spinal border and flair outward, slowly gliding along the rib cage. Come back to center, placing thumbs ¼ to ½ inches below previous position and stroke outward. In this fashion, work your way down the back.

2. *Using the back of the hand(s).* For a lighter stroke, stroke along the spinal column and outward along the ribs. You can use a second hand for leverage and support.

3. *Using the knuckles.* You can stroke slowly and deeply with the knuckles, moving horizontally and vertically along the lower back. Experiment with what feels the best to you.

4. *Using the four fingers and palm.* With the flat of four fingers and the palm, stroke up and down along the sides of the spinal column (go up only as far as comfort allows). Stroke back and forth out along the ribs.

Helpful Hints: Experiment and do what is easiest for you. The next time your lower back aches from tension or weakness you will know what to do. Simply stroke it.

Avoid applying direct pressure on the spine. It is best if you work *both* sides of the spine.

Beneficial Effects: Increases circulation in the lower back.

Soothes and warms as it relieves excessive muscular tension.

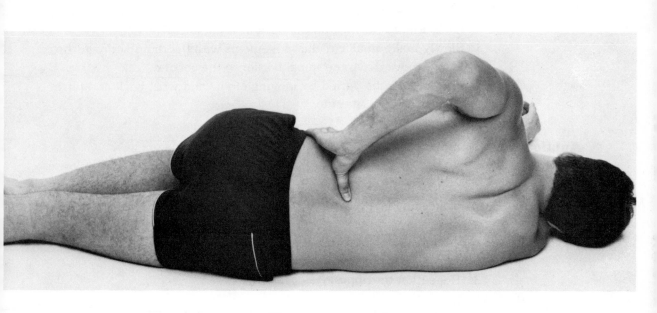

THE BACK: APPLICATION 5
FRICTION

Position: Lying on your side for the lower back.
Sitting for the upper back.
Using the thumb and four fingers.

Application: *Treating the lower back*

1. Lie on your left side. Bend your right leg, bringing your knee to your chest.
2. With bent elbow, bring your right hand back to the center of your back. Place it as high up the back as is comfortable.
3. Slowly make small circular movements with the thumb or fingertips as you move down the spinal border to the coccyx.
4. Pressure can be varied by moving elbow and wrist back and forth. Repeat on opposite side.

Application: *Treating the upper back*

1. While sitting, bring your right arm across your chest to opposite shoulder, elbow pointing outward, so that the right hand is able to make contact along the spine.
2. Using the flats of two or three fingertips, make deep circles along the spinal column, in between the spine and shoulder blade, and across the shoulder blade itself.
3. Repeat on the opposite side.

Helpful Hints: It is best to treat *both* sides of the back.

Stretch out your shoulders by rolling them afterward: lift shoulders and draw them back. Drop them back down and bring them back around. This will make a circle. Do a couple to relieve any acquired shoulder tension.

Follow your normal breathing patterns. If you find a sensitive spot while working your way down the back, deeply exhale and hold the spot.

The more you practice this move, the stronger your fingers become.

Beneficial Effects: Stimulates circulation and metabolic interchange.
Relieves stiffness in the back as it redistributes lactic acid build-up.

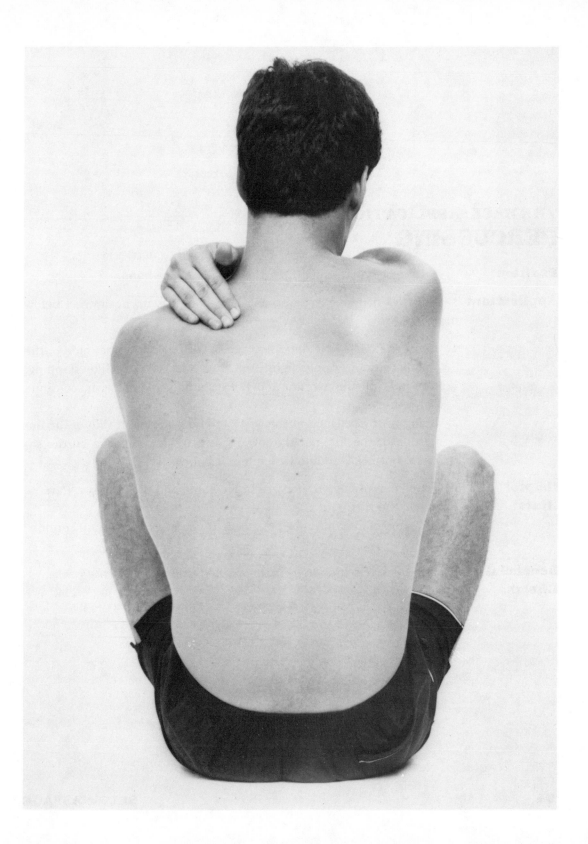

THE BACK: APPLICATION 6
PERCUSSING

Position: Sitting or lying, using the fist or the flat of the hand.

Application: Start by bringing your arm(s) back behind you, positioned below the rib cage.

1. *Using the flat of the hand.* Pat the lower back on either side of the spinal column. Apply lightly at first. This is a lot like slapping. Continue on the sacrum and buttocks and, if you wish, continue down the legs.
2. *Using your fist.* Bend at the wrist and with the palm side of the flat portion of the fist, pat the lower back. Again, continue on the sacrum, buttocks, and down the legs if you wish.

Helpful Hints: Avoid percussing on the vertebral column and the kidneys. Percuss *lightly* on the ribs.

Stop and shake out your hands when you are tired before continuing.

Beneficial Effects: Stimulates circulation as it aids in the relief of stiff, tense backs.

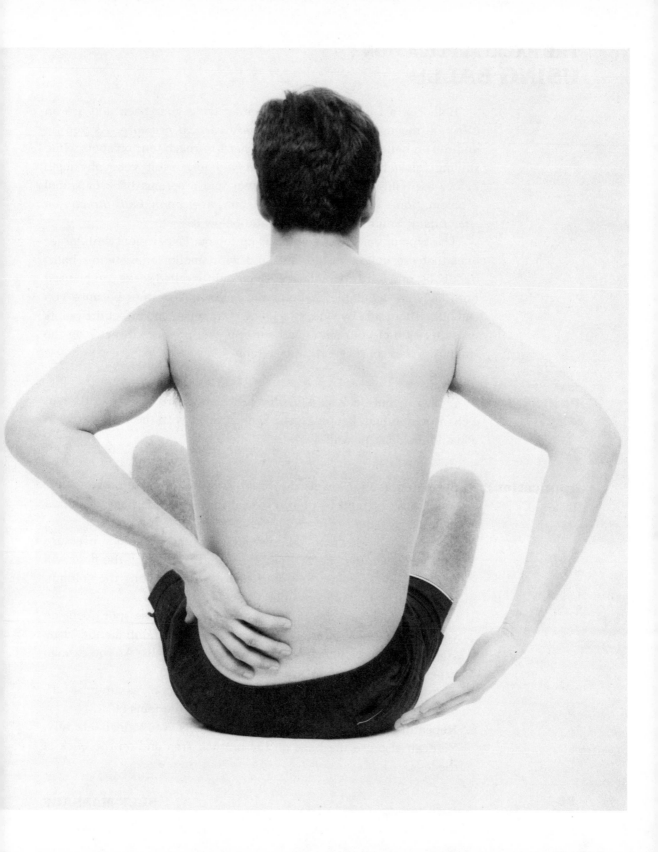

THE BACK: APPLICATION 7
USING BALLS

Balls can act as a pair of hands massaging your back and are an effective means for applying *stationary vertical pressure*. As you lie and roll on balls you can locate those hard-to-reach tension spots while staying relaxed. However, I caution you to consult your physician before applying balls if you have ever had a serious back or spinal problem. Some sensitivity is normal, but *never apply balls directly on site of pain*. You may work above and below it.

The type of balls that you use is up to you. Experiment with larger ones that are hollow inside, and also with smaller ones: tennis balls, handballs, and hard spongy ones. Even tightly rolled socks can be used until balls are available. I prefer the larger hollow ones because you can place them side by side, straddling your spine, and affect the points on either side of your spine without applying pressure directly on the spinous process of the vertebral column.

Position: Lying on your back on a flat and preferably hard surface. Sitting in a chair or standing, keeping your back straight with the balls between you and the chair or wall.

Application: 1. Beginning as high up as the base of the cranium, a pair of balls equal in size should be placed so that they are straddling the spinal column.
2. Inch the balls down to the sacrum, working the major pressure points (refer to the chart). Bent knees and feet flat on the floor will give you leverage and help you move the balls along the column, or you can sit up and reposition the balls.
3. Once the balls have been placed on a point or tense spot, focus on your breathing. With arms and shoulders relaxed, inhale and bring your breath to the points being affected by the balls. As you exhale, expel the tension out. Continue to the next spot.
4. The recommended amount of time per spot is a maximum of 10 minutes. Follow your instincts—you know what feels best.
5. Repeat the entire process by moving the balls ¼ to ½ inch laterally. You can also use the balls on the buttock area and on the back of the legs.

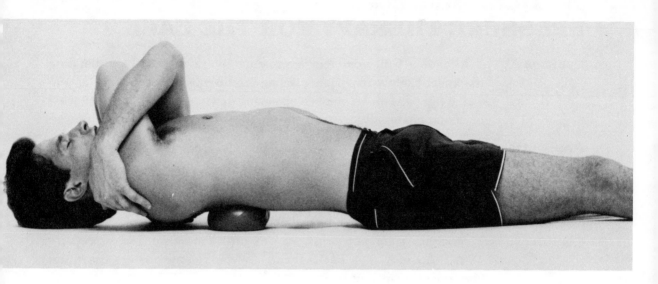

Variations: As you apply the balls to pressure points and tense spots, experiment with some movement. Move slowly, be aware of your breath, as you center your attention on the area being affected by the balls.

1. Inhale, lifting arm(s) above your head. Exhale as you hold the position; inhale, arm(s) up across your chest and exhale down. Now breathe normally.
2. Experiment and explore with movement by bending your knees and using different arm positions.

Be creative and listen to your body. You will know when you have done enough.

Helpful Hints: It is best to work with two balls at a time. If you have trouble stabilizing the balls, try wrapping them in a towel: place the balls in a towel and fold the towel over them. Twist the towel around the balls at the center and at the ends. If the towel is long enough you should be able to move the balls down the spine by holding on to the ends of the towel.

Beneficial Effects: Redistributes lactic acid build-up (which is a cause of muscle stiffness).

Relieves tense, fatigued areas of the back.

Works the inner and outer Urinary Bladder meridian, releasing energy blocks.

The Back   **97**

PRESSURE THERAPY FOR THE BACK

Position: Standing with your feet approximately 12 inches apart, bending the knees slightly for balance, using the thumbs of both hands; or you can apply balls to the points while lying down.

Treat bilaterally.

Application: 1. With arms drawn back, simultaneously place the balls of both thumbs along either side of the spinal column. Place them as high up as comfort and freedom of movement allow.

2. Focus on your breath. As you inhale, place the thumbs. As you exhale, draw your elbows back and lean back into your thumbs, applying *stationary pressure*. The direction of the thumb pressure is deep into your back. Inhale as you release the pressure and straighten up your back.

3. Move your thumbs down the Urinary Bladder channel one vertebral space at a time, continuing down the column to the sacrum. Continue along the points in the buttock as you work along either side of the sacrum out toward the hipbones.

4. Rest a minute and shake out your hands. Repeat the application, working ½ to 1 inch lateral to the previous position. You will have applied pressure on two imaginary lines on each side of the column as you go down your back. This is working the inner and outer Urinary Bladder meridian.

Helpful Hints: The timing of the pressure and release is up to you. It is recommended that you hold the more sensitive points longer. For general timing, exhale and apply pressure to the count of 5 and inhale and release to the count of 3.

There should be little or no exertion, as you allow your body weight and gravity to do the work. Just lean into your thumbs—there's no need to use muscle. Leaning is minimal, going back only as far as your balance and comfort allow.

Avoid applying pressure on *painful* points. Instead, just hold these points, and work above and below the site of pain.

Beneficial Effects: Releases lower back tension and tension in the legs.

Releases blocks within the Urinary Bladder channel and gall bladder points in buttocks.

Improves circulation and helps to maintain good health.

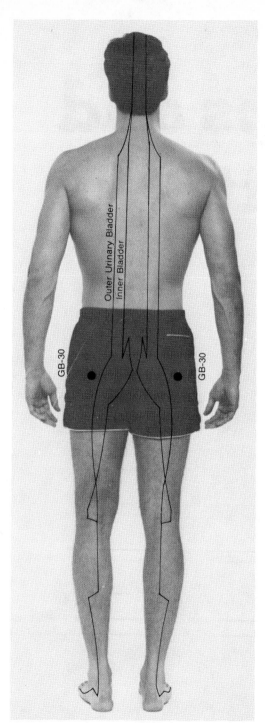

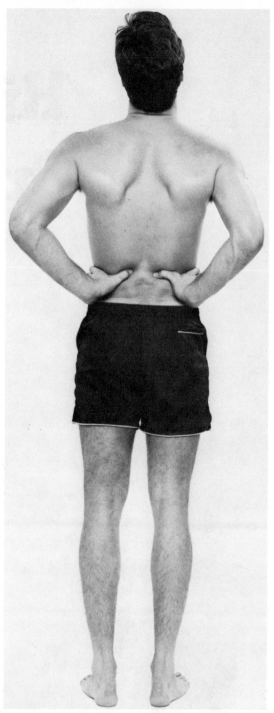

Major Points: All Urinary Bladder points are to be affected in the back.
(GB-30) Gall Bladder point in the buttocks.

The Back

Hips and
Buttocks

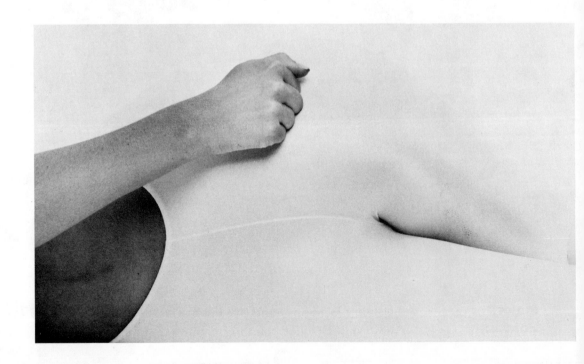

KNUCKLE-STROKE

Position: Lying on your side (starting on either side) with outside leg slightly bent, bringing knee toward chest. Use knuckles and palm of one hand.

Application:

1. Lying on either side, you will work the outside buttock and hip with the outside hand.
2. Make a fist, and with your knuckles begin on the edge of the hip-bone (inferior iliac crest).
3. Stroke diagonally across the buttock (gluteal muscle) toward the coccyx. By doing this you will be going with the grain of muscle fiber. Continue across and down toward the underside of the buttocks.
4. Release your fist and stroke back up with the palm of the hand.
5. Repeat 10 times slowly. Change sides, working opposite hip and buttock.

Helpful Hints: This is an excellent movement to do with deep breathing: exhale as you knuckle down and across buttocks. Inhale deeply as you stroke up. Pressure is firm but comfortable, allowing for bony protuberances. Continue this movement on the outer thighs.

Beneficial Effects: May aid in breaking down adipose tissue (fat).
Locally stimulates circulation and metabolic interchange.
Helps relieve stiffness in hip.

HIPS AND BUTTOCKS: APPLICATION 2
VIBRATION

Position: Lying on your side (starting on either side) with outside leg slightly bent, bringing the knee toward the chest.

Use four fingers of one hand.

Application: 1. Lying on either side, with your hand you can vibrate the hip and buttock region. You will be applying horizontal vibration.

2. Begin on the upper edge of the hipbone (inferior iliac crest).

3. Vibrate horizontally for 2 seconds and release. Move hand down. Repeat. Continue down to hip joint.

4. Also vibrate horizontally along the buttock, moving your hand toward the coccyx and down to the underside of the buttocks.

5. Repeat on other side.

Helpful Hints: If you have any problem executing the move, refer to the movements section of the chapter on self-massage technique.

Do not remain too long on one spot, but vibrate for at least 2 seconds.

Remember to keep shoulders and arms relaxed.

Beneficial Effects: Maintaining circulation and tissue fluid interchange.

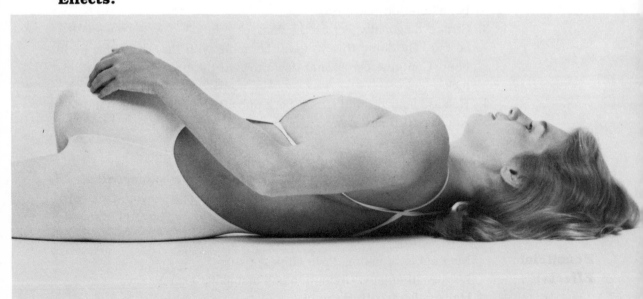

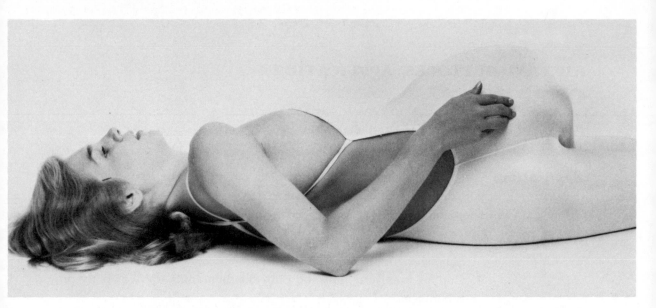

HIPS AND BUTTOCKS: APPLICATION 3
FRICTION

Position: Lying on your side (starting on either side) with outside leg slightly bent, bringing the knee toward the chest. Use four strong fingers and the palm, or thumb if necessary, for leverage.

Application: 1. Beginning at the sacrum (middle lower back) make deep, circular movements with the balls of the fingertips. Travel outward along the iliac crest (hipbone).
2. Continue to the edge of the hipbone and travel down around the hip joint making smaller circles.
3. Work back up toward the coccyx and begin across the buttocks, separating the fibers of the gluteal muscle.
4. Work the entire area 5 minutes. Change sides and repeat.

Helpful Hints: Remember to make smaller circles around bony protuberances and larger circles on body of muscle.

Larger circles can be made with the whole hand while smaller circles are best done with four fingers.

Beneficial Effects: Stimulates circulation and tissue fluid interchange.

Maintains joint mobility and muscle power.

HIPS AND BUTTOCKS: APPLICATION 4
CUPPING

Position: Using one hand while lying on your side.
Using two hands while standing.

Application: Of all the percussion movements, cupping is the easiest to use on your hips and buttocks. You can do it while lying on your side, with one hand, or while standing, using both hands.

1. Position your hand(s) in a half fist with the fingers together. Your hand(s) should look like a cup.
2. Cup all over your hips and buttocks, lightening up over bony protuberances.
3. Percuss each side 5 to 10 times.

Helpful Hints: Keep shoulders relaxed.
As with all percussion movements, be careful not to bruise.

Beneficial Effects: Stimulates circulation and disperses metabolic waste products.

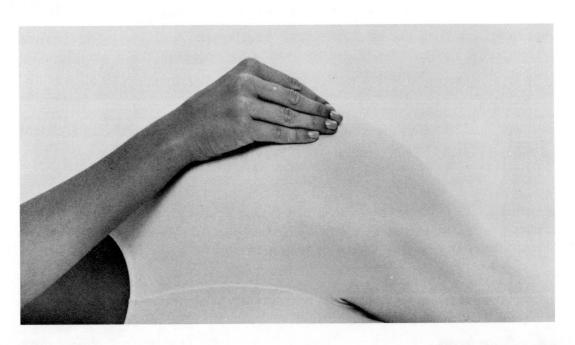

The Legs

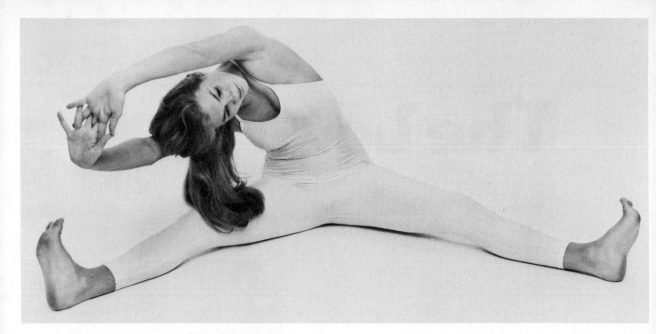

THE LEGS: APPLICATION 1
LEG STRETCHES

Position: Sitting on the floor, bed, or mat.

Application: 1. Sitting up with your back straight, spread your legs outward. This should not be painful, but don't be afraid to stretch.
2. Interlock your fingers and invert them as you stretch your arms above your head.
3. Inhale deeply, and as you exhale let your breath take you over your left leg as far as you can go. As you stretch, the head and torso should remain full front so that you are not twisting your body.
4. Hold the position following normal breathing patterns. Inhale and then exhale, pushing yourself down a little further. Return to an upright position.
5. Repeat on the right side.
6. Repeat as you stretch forward out from the center of your body, directing your head and chest toward the floor. Stretch yourself out as far as possible.

Helpful Hints: The stretch begins from the lower back, keeping the back as straight as possible.

Beneficial Effects: Stretches out the meridian channels.
Stretches and strengthens the back muscles.

STROKING

Position: Sitting or lying with leg muscles relaxed, using the balls of the fingertips of one or both hands.

Application: 1. This is a simple movement following the direction of the muscle fibers as you stroke up and down the leg.

            2. To facilitate circulation, firm strokes are directed toward the heart.

            3. You can begin anywhere on either leg, using one hand or both. Try it with one hand while lying down with your knees bent. Or, lie on either side and work inner and outer legs, bending your knees accordingly so that you have easy access to different parts of your legs.

            4. Try stroking with the knee or heel of one foot, up and down the leg, while lying down. Varying amounts of pressure can be applied by flexing and extending your ankle as you stroke.

Helpful Hints: The whole leg can be massaged while sitting in a chair, but remember to keep the shoulders and arms relaxed.

          Follow normal breathing patterns.

          This is a great massage movement to practice while relaxing in a warm bath.

Beneficial Effects: Warms and soothes tired aching legs, increasing circulation and lymphatic drainage.

          Stroking is a good move for exploring your body. Discover your sensitive, blocked spots and work them out.

          This feels especially nice on the legs if you have been sitting all day.

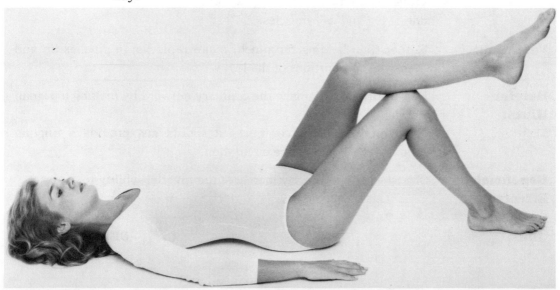

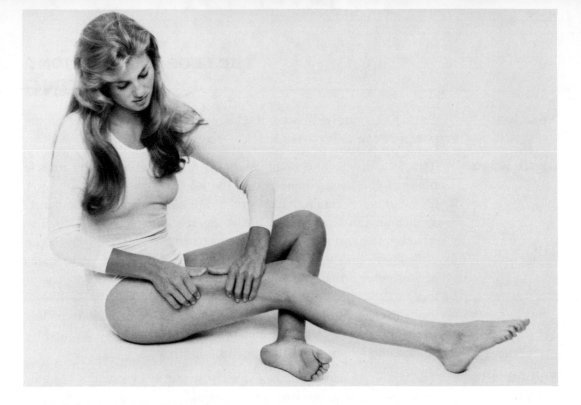

THE LEGS: APPLICATION 3
THE PINCH

Position: Sitting or lying with knees bent, using palms and opposing four fingers or thumbs and opposing four fingers.

Application: 1. This is to be applied on the fleshier areas of the legs.
2. Gently hold the body of the muscle, pulling slightly.
3. Hold and release, gliding off the muscle.
4. Travel up and down the leg, working front, back, inside, and outside of leg and calf muscles.

Variation: Rather than holding the pinch, make rapid, large pinches up and down the fleshier portions of the leg.

Helpful Hints: Be careful not to damage the capillary network by making too small a pinch.

The pinch should never hurt—it should just provide a tingling sensation as it stimulates the circulation.

Beneficial Effects: Stretches and indirectly increases the muscles' ability to contract.

ROLLING

Position: Sitting with your knees bent: in a chair, on a bed, or on the floor, using the palms and heels of both hands.

Application: 1. Beginning on the calf of your leg, place your palms on either side of the calf just below the knee. Palms are placed on the muscle and are straddling the bone. Fingers will be pointing outward from the body.

        2. With alternating palms, roll the muscle body back and forth around the bone. Work up and down the calf with a rolling, rhythmic motion.

        3. Roll both calves and thighs. When applying rolling to your thighs the fingers will be pointing down. Allow 2 to 5 minutes for each calf and thigh.

Helpful Hints: This movement is similar to rolling a ball of clay between your hands.

    Your shoulders are to be down and relaxed.

Beneficial Effects: Friends of mine who do distance running like to use this move when their legs start to cramp. Five minutes of rolling helps restore muscle strength and redistribute lactic acid build-up.

    Relieves muscle spasm in calves.

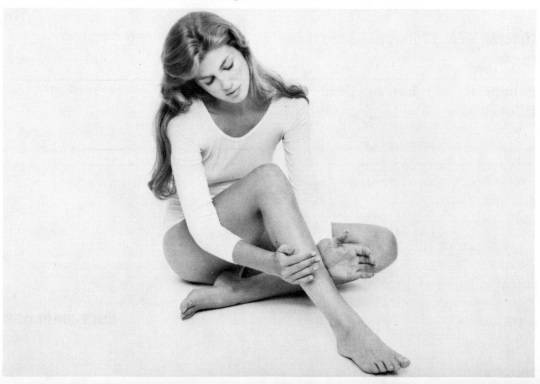

THE LEGS: APPLICATION 5
PETRISSAGE

Position: Sitting with all muscles relaxed, using both hands or just one.

Application:
1. Place both hands side by side so they are horizontal to the thigh.
2. With hands straddling the muscle body, pick up, roll, and push the muscle body with one hand as you pull with the other.
3. This is done in an alternating pattern as your hands glide vertically along the muscle body without breaking contact.
4. The calf can be massaged with one hand gliding up and down; as you roll, squeeze and pull the muscle between the thumb and fingers.

Helpful Hints: Keep shoulders relaxed by centering on your breathing.

Beneficial Effects: Increases circulation and disperses metabolic waste products.

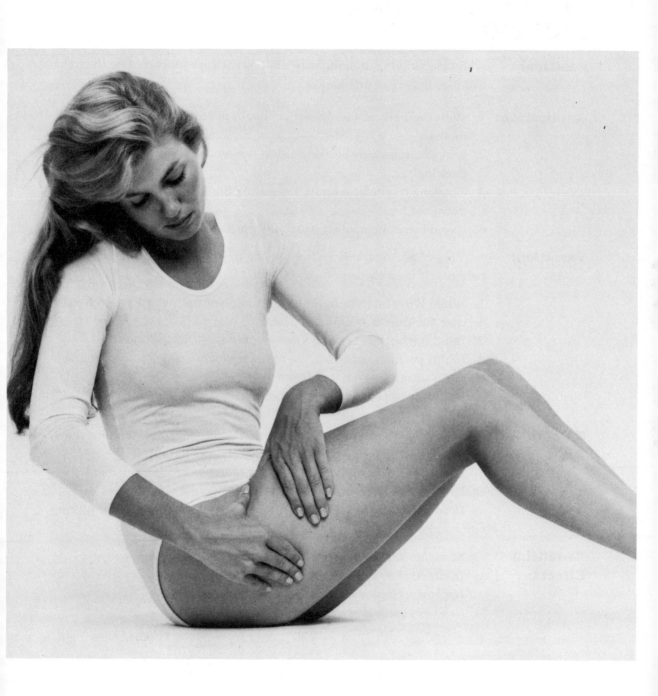

THE LEGS: APPLICATION 6
FRICTION

Position: Sitting or lying, making sure that muscles are relaxed. Use the palm and four fingers of one hand.

Application: 1. With the balls of the fingertips, begin making small circular movements.
2. Larger circles can be done using the whole hand. It's like circular stroking.
3. Go along the muscle body, separating the fibers as you work up and down the leg.
4. Avoid breaking contact with skin's surface.

Variation: This is an excellent technique for the elderly and for bedridden patients. It is soothing and easy to do.

1. While lying on your side, bring inside leg up toward your chest so that the knee is comfortably bent.
2. Bend the outside leg and knee slightly.
3. In this position apply friction to the inside of one leg and the outside of the other.
4. Roll over to your other side and repeat.

Helpful Hints: Friction is especially good around joint capsules (ankles, hips, knees). When applying to these areas make smaller circles.

Remember to keep your shoulders relaxed, and if your hands tire, shake them out from time to time.

If your hands are weak, this movement can be applied by placing one hand over the other.

Beneficial Effects: Stretches and strengthens muscle fibers.
Is effective in breaking down scar tissue.
Improves circulation and tissue fluid interchange.

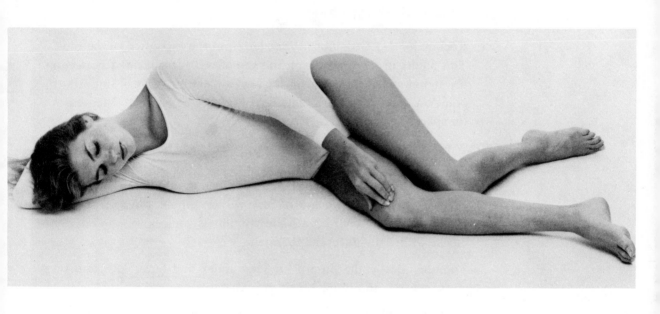

THE LEGS: APPLICATION 7
PRESSURE THERAPY
FOR THE LEGS AND FEET

Position: When sitting you can use thumbs, palms, elbows, and fingers. When lying down you can use the heel of your foot. Treat bilaterally.

Application: Consider the leg as having two sides: inner and outer. The inner is usually lighter with less hair, whereas the outer is darker with more hair. Within the inner legs are the Spleen, Pancreas, Liver, and Kidney pathways. Within the outer legs are the Stomach, Gall Bladder and Urinary Bladder pathways.

1. *Recommended Direction:* Work leg from the hip down to the toes. The points in the feet are on the top of each foot located between the metatarsals (refer to chart). There is only one very important point on the soles of the feet, Ki-1 (kidney 1). Refer to the charts for specific points.

2. Work effortlessly by leaning into the points whenever possible. Let your body weight and the force of gravity do the work. Synchronize your breathing with the application: exhale as you apply *stationary vertical pressure* to a count of 5, and then inhale and release to a count of 3. Bring your breath into motion as you release the energy blocks within the different channels.

3. *Thumbs:* Use your thumbs on your inner and outer legs and on your feet (i.e., thumbing down the calf).

4. *Fingers:* Apply pressure with the fingers on the back of the legs. This is easily done while lying down with knees in upright position toward your chest. With fingers of both hands slightly curled, start by the buttocks and work down to the knees along the Urinary Bladder meridian.

5. *Elbows and Palms:* These are good for applying pressure on the inner and outer legs. Lean your weight into the area being affected. When using the elbow, try a soft elbow penetration and then flex your arm for a harder elbow penetration.

6. *Heel of the Foot:* While lying down you can affect the points on the inner and outer legs. For the inner leg, bend and evert the leg to be

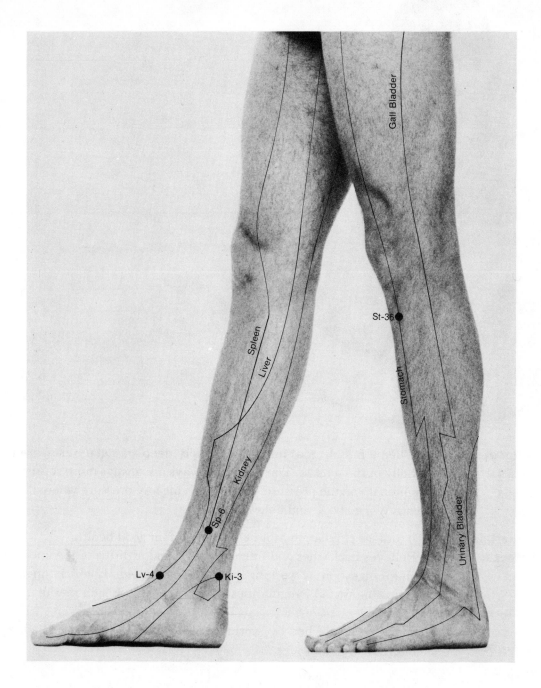

treated, letting it lie in a comfortable, outward position. Apply pressure with the opposite heel. Treat the outer leg by turning the bent knee inward as you slightly invert the leg. Different amounts of pressure can be applied by flexing ankles and pointing toes.

The Legs

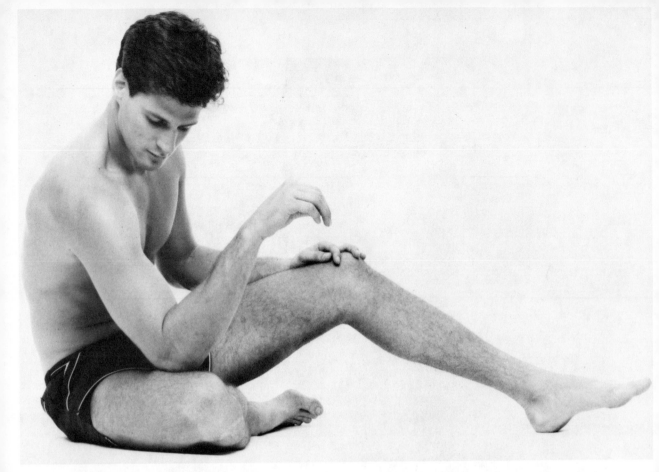

Helpful Hints: When a muscle goes into spasm, apply deep *stationary pressure* to the belly of the muscle. The inner pathways are always more sensitive, so lighten up on the pressure. Avoid applying any pressure where there is pain. Work above and below it.

Beneficial Effects: Improves circulation as it helps to maintain good health.

Relieves backaches and fatigue in legs, and arthritis of the knee.

Helps digestion by working the Stomach, Spleen, Liver channels.

Helps menstrual irregularities by working the Spleen meridian on the inner leg.

Relieves headaches by working the Stomach and Gall Bladder channels on the outer legs.

Major Points:

St-36	Stomach
Lv-4	Liver
Sp-6	Spleen
Ki-1 & 3	Kidney

SELF-MASSAGE

The Feet

FOOT MASSAGE is a part of the science of reflexology, or zone therapy, which has its roots in ancient Chinese culture. This is a part of a system of reflex points, or zones, that are also located on the ears, eyes, and hands. These zones correspond to the organs, nerves, and glands within the body, as illustrated in the foot chart. When massaging the foot, feel for tight muscles and tendons, hollow spaces and nodules, and listen for cracking sounds. Work these sensitive areas, releasing tension as you stimulate the reflex points, relieving energy imbalance. I have provided you with a few good basic moves. If you have further interest in the science of reflexology, there are several books out on the subject that you can consult such as *The Foot Book* by Devaki Berkson.

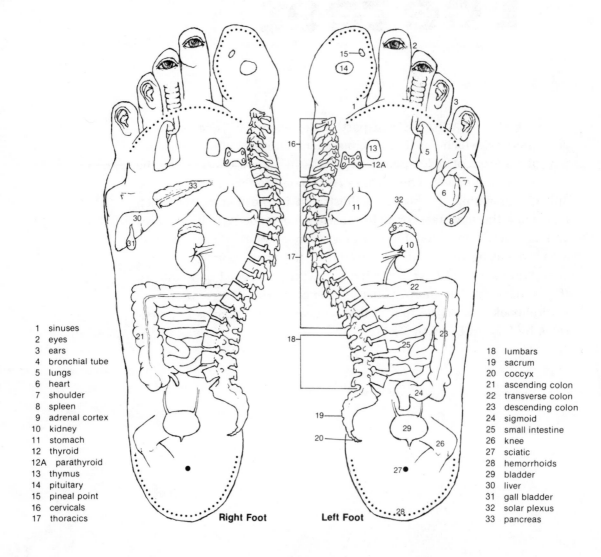

1 sinuses	
2 eyes	
3 ears	
4 bronchial tube	
5 lungs	
6 heart	
7 shoulder	
8 spleen	18 lumbars
9 adrenal cortex	19 sacrum
10 kidney	20 coccyx
11 stomach	21 ascending colon
12 thyroid	22 transverse colon
12A parathyroid	23 descending colon
13 thymus	24 sigmoid
14 pituitary	25 small intestine
15 pineal point	26 knee
16 cervicals	27 sciatic
17 thoracics	28 hemorrhoids
	29 bladder
	30 liver
	31 gall bladder
	32 solar plexus
	33 pancreas

Right Foot   **Left Foot**

FOOT AND TOE STRETCHES

Position: Sitting or lying down.

Application: *Foot Stretches:*

1. Point your toes toward your nose. Hold 10 to 20 seconds as you stretch out the Achilles tendons.
2. Point your toes down, stretching them for 10 to 20 seconds.
3. Point your toes inward toward each other and hold 10 to 20 seconds.
4. Point your toes outward and hold 10 to 20 seconds.
5. Shake out your feet. These stretches can be repeated 5 times.
6. Make circles with your ankles, 3 times to the right and 3 times to the left.
7. Try flexing your feet against resistance. For example: flex your foot against your hand or flex one foot against the other. Be creative and experiment.

Application: *Toe Stretches.* Try these stretches while sitting comfortable with one leg crossed over the opposite thigh so that the foot is hanging freely.

Extension:

1. Anchor your palm at the base of your toes on the top of the foot.
2. Curl your fingers around and over the toes so that your fingertips are positioned on the sole of the foot at the base of the toes.
3. Extend and stretch your toes by moving your hand forward. Your fingers will be pushing your toes toward the heel of the foot.

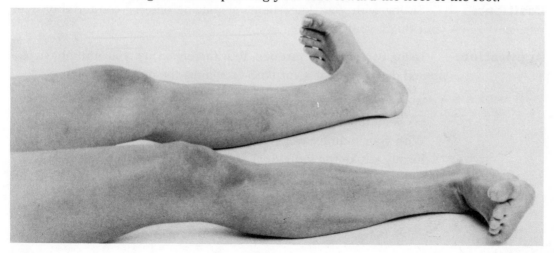

The Feet

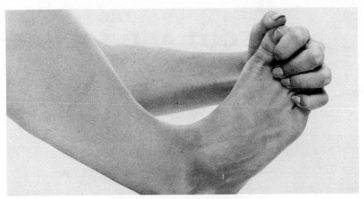

Application: Flexion:

1. Anchor your palm at the base of your toes on the sole of your foot.
2. Curl your fingers around and over the toes so that your fingertips are positioned on top of the foot at the base of the toes.
3. Flex and stretch your toes by moving your hand forward toward your knee. The angle of pressure is down into the foot.
4. Repeat both extension and flexion on the opposite foot.

Beneficial Effects: The foot stretches are good for fallen arches and abused feet, by stretching out and strengthening the tendons.

Toe stretches are good for tired feet and stimulate the reflex points located on the feet.

THE FEET: APPLICATION 2
STROKING

Position: Sitting with your knee bent, or placing one leg comfortably over your thigh, your foot free.

Application: Using two hands or just one, four fingers or just your thumb, stroke up and down the foot going with or against the muscle fibers.

1. Work the top portion of the foot, molding the fingers on and in between the tendons and down to the toes.
2. With your thumbs, work the tops and bottoms and sides of the toes. Firmly stroke the individual joint spaces of each toe.
3. Extend the foot and work the top of the ankle. Flex the foot and work the heel and Achilles tendon.
4. With your thumbs or four fingers on each side, stroke around the ankle bone.

5. On the sole of the foot, stroke with your thumbs while you hold your foot in your hands. Stroke vertically up and down the foot. While alternating your thumbs, stroke horizontally across the sole.

Variation: If you are too tired to sit, bedridden, or just lying down, try stroking one foot with the *heel* of the other foot.

1. Anchor your heel on the sole of the opposite foot. Push and stroke back and forth. Continue in this fashion on the top of the foot and around the ankles.
2. With the toes of the giving foot upright, place the heel of the receiving foot in between the big toe and second toe. Stroke up and down on the Achilles tendon as you flex and extend your toes. Try to work your Achilles tendon in between the other toes too. This is a good stretch for the toes.

Beneficial Effects: Deep application stimulates the reflex points.
This exercise is warm and soothing, feels great on those tired, aching feet.

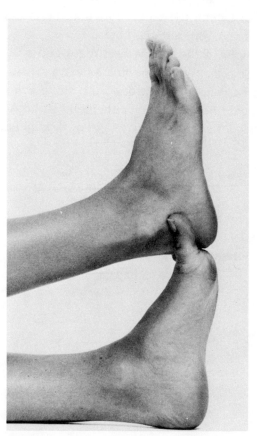

THE FEET: APPLICATION 3
FRICTION

Position: Sitting with your foot flat on the floor, or with one leg crossed over the opposite thigh so that your foot is resting on the thigh; using your strongest fingers or just your thumbs.

Application:
1. Make small, deep circles, affecting the tissue underneath the skin's surface.
2. Be creative and experiment by flexing and extending your foot in different directions as you apply friction. When massaging the ankle, extend the toes, stretching the muscle. As you massage the ligaments, separate the fibers.
3. The sole of the foot is best massaged with your thumbs, making deep circles. When you find an extra sensitive spot, work it out.
4. It is easiest to work around the ankle using the index and middle fingers of both hands on either side of the Achilles tendon. Massage both sides simultaneously as you work up and down and around the ankle.

Helpful Hints: When you massage the top of your foot, work in the direction of your ankle. When you massage the sole of your foot, work toward the toes.

Beneficial Effects: Breaks up waste deposits.
Stimulates the reflex points, affecting all body systems.

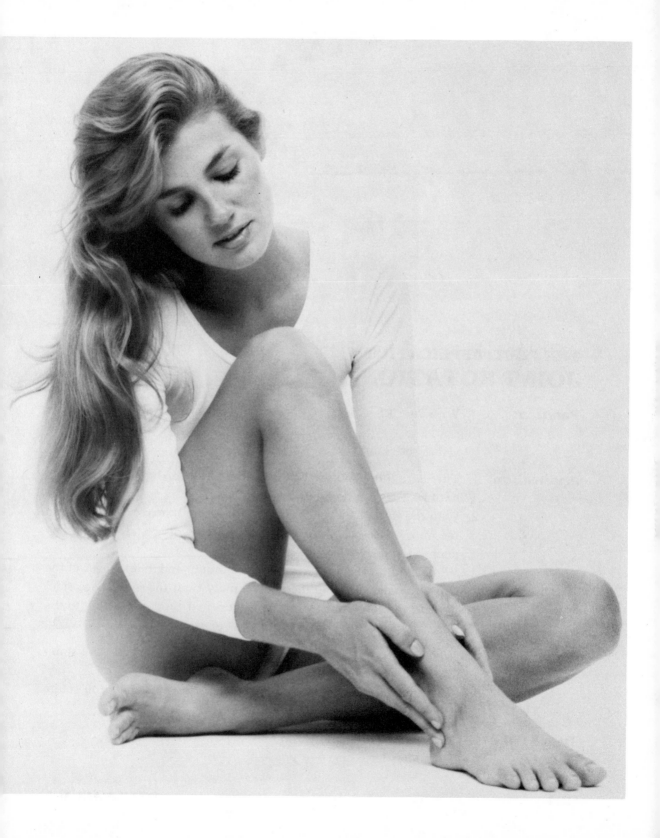

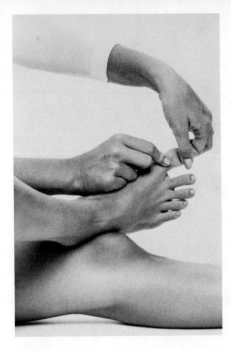

THE FEET: APPLICATION 4
JOINT ROTATION

Position: With your knee bent, place your leg comfortably over the opposite thigh.

Using both hands.

Application: 1. There are three joints in each toe, except for the big toe, which only has two, that can be rotated sideways.
2. With the thumb and index finger of one hand, hold firmly between the joint spaces of the toes. You will be holding and rotating one joint at a time.
3. While holding one joint space use the thumb and index finger of the opposite hand to rotate the joint. Simply twist the joint space sideways to the left and then to the right 3 to 4 times. Move on to the next joint space and repeat.

Helpful Hints: When rotating the first joints at the base of the foot, you will stabilize by holding the ball of the foot.

As with the fingers, you stabilize below the joint while you rotate above it.

Beneficial Effects: Maintains joint mobility and muscle power.
Stimulates local nerve response.

PERCUSSING

Position: Sitting in a relaxed position with one leg over the opposite thigh so that the foot is hanging freely.

Application: 1. While supporting the foot with one hand, slap the sole of the foot with the opposite hand. Slap with the flat portion of the fingers vigorously for 15 to 20 seconds or until your hands get tired.

              2. Shake out your hand and apply to the opposite foot.

Variation: While lying down, try slapping the soles of your feet together. Instead of clapping your hands you are clapping your feet. Clap 5 to 10 times and shake out.

Helpful Hints: This is good to do before and after other applications to the feet.

Beneficial Effects: Stimulates the reflex zones to all body systems.

        Great for tired feet when you have been wearing high heels or have been on your feet all day.

        Warms up those cold feet.

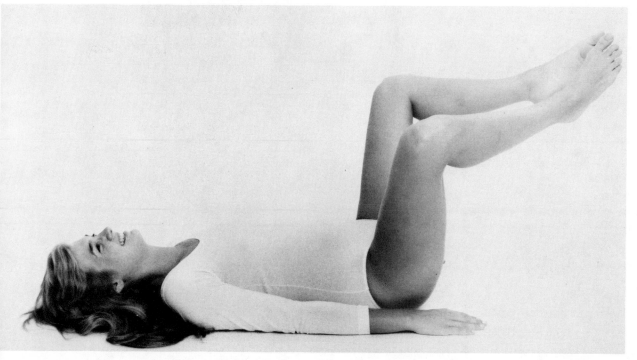

The Feet